Advance Praise for
Race and Excellence: My Dialogue With Chester Pierce

"At once deeply intimate and broad in scope, Ezra Griffith's project to capture the life and accomplishments of Chester Pierce shares profound personal reflections on life, race, psychiatry, and beyond by both men. Nearly 25 years after its first publication, *Race and Excellence* remains a sensitive, insightful, and impactful contribution to understandings of race, privilege, and profession at this pivotal time of psychiatry's—and society's—reckoning with dismantling structures and institutions of racism. The life and lessons of Dr. Pierce shared through the lens of his accomplishments and choices about where to focus his extraordinary talents and energy challenge us all to be both deliberate and aspirational in our lives, work, relationships, and commitments."

Rebecca Weintraub Brendel, M.D., J.D., DFAPA, President-Elect, American Psychiatric Association

"In *Race and Excellence: My Dialogue With Chester Pierce,* Ezra Griffith deftly combines elements of biography and autobiography to present us with a picture of the complex man that was Chester Pierce. Most readers may know that Pierce was a famous Black psychiatrist, but it is likely that few are aware of the breadth and depth of his unique personal and professional experiences. Here we learn about many of Pierce's singular accomplishments, including being the first Black player on a segregated college football field south of the Mason-Dixon line, the first Black psychiatrist to become director and president of the American Board of Psychiatry and Neurology, and the founding president of the Black Psychiatrists of America. In response to probing from Griffith that is both gentle and persistent, Pierce discusses everything from his important research on extreme environments such as Antarctica to his consultation with the creators of Sesame Street to his observations about the microaggressions endured day in and day out by Blacks and other minorities. In the process of their conversations, Griffith uncovers not just facts about Pierce's life but also subtleties in his personality and strategies that helped him either avoid or overcome obstacles to his success. This well-written book would certainly be valuable even if it only documented the trailblazing life of Chester Pierce. I believe it is even more important, however, for what it reveals about how one might rise above an environment of tension and conflict to create a life of excellence and achievement."

Larry R. Faulkner, M.D., President and CEO, American Board of Psychiatry and Neurology

"In his biography of African American Harvard psychiatrist Chester Pierce, Ezra Griffith, a gifted storyteller and psychiatrist, provides the reader a window into the life of a great man at close psychological range. Born in 1927, Pierce was influenced by the quiet support of his mother and the entrepreneurial determination of his father, once a shoe shiner in Harlem. By age 25, he had graduated from Harvard Medical School. Pierce was an intellectual with wide-ranging scholarship and professional achievements, including consultancy to *Sesame Street* and NASA. However, he was not immune to the racial affronts ever present in the United States. Such encounters highlighted the fabric of racial prejudice—the microtraumas and macrotraumas—against Blacks. He cofounded the professional association Black Psychiatrists of America as a pathway for positive impact. Griffith writes, "I never wanted just to tell Chet's story; I wanted to work his story out, to measure it, to try it on, to figure out which parts are good for me and for other blacks so earnestly seeking heroes." Griffith most certainly achieves this goal. *Race and Excellence* is as contemporary in its relevance today as it was when first issued in 1998."

Shoba Sreenivasan, Ph.D., Adjunct Professor, Keck USC School of Medicine, Institute of Psychiatry, Law and Behavioral Sciences; Forensic Psychologist—Forensic Services Division, California Department of State Hospitals

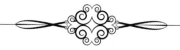

RACE AND EXCELLENCE
My Dialogue With Chester Pierce

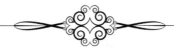

RACE AND EXCELLENCE
My Dialogue With Chester Pierce

EZRA E.H. GRIFFITH, M.D.

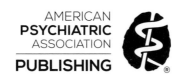

If you wish to buy 50 or more copies of the same title, please go to www.appi.org/specialdiscounts for more information.

Copyright © 2023 American Psychiatric Association Publishing
ALL RIGHTS RESERVED
Reprint edition with bonus material; University of Iowa Press edition published 1998

Manufactured in the United States of America on acid-free paper
25 24 23 22 21   5 4 3 2 1

American Psychiatric Association Publishing
800 Maine Avenue SW
Suite 900
Washington, DC 20024-2812
www.appi.org

Library of Congress Cataloging-in-Publication Data
A CIP record is available from the Library of Congress.

British Library Cataloguing in Publication Data
A CIP record is available from the British Library.

To Véronique and Pierre, who have made
Brigitte and me proud antecedents of their stories, and to
Vincent and Ermie, who started it all.

CONTENTS

About the Author

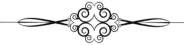

Ezra Griffith is Professor Emeritus of Psychiatry and African-American Studies at Yale University. He was born in Barbados and received his undergraduate education at Harvard College and his medical education in France. He was on the faculty at the Yale School of Medicine from 1977 to 2016. During that time, he held several administrative leadership positions, including Director of the Connecticut Mental Health Center. He taught classes on Black autobiographies in the Faculty of Arts and Sciences.

Dr. Griffith is a former president of the Black Psychiatrists of America, the American Orthopsychiatric Association, and the American Academy of Psychiatry and the Law. In 2001, the Morehouse School of Medicine conferred on him an honorary Doctor of Science degree. He served for 20 years as editor of the *Journal of the American Academy of Psychiatry and the Law*. In 2010, the American Psychiatric Association presented him its Isaac Ray Award for distinguished achievements in forensic psychiatry.

Dr. Griffith has published widely in the subdisciplines of forensic psychiatry and cultural psychiatry. He has written most recently on ethics and matters of diversity, inclusion, and belonging. He has proposed human dignity as a significant factor in rendering social spaces more therapeutic. He is the author of *Belonging, Therapeutic Landscapes, and Networks* (Routledge, 2018), the editor of *Ethics Challenges in Forensic Psychiatry and Psychology Practice* (Columbia University Press, 2018), and a coeditor of *Black Mental Health* (American Psychiatric Publishing, 2019).

Preface

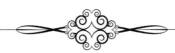

Over the past two decades, I have been a serious student of the Black life. I have been unceasingly curious about how African American men and women tell the stories of their lives, recount their successes and failures, explain their way of coping with everyday trauma, and joyously announce their celebrations. Such storytelling has held special fascination for me because I have viewed it as a window on thinking and problem-solving by African Americans. Specialists from other disciplines have been quick to see the literary, historical, and cultural significance of the Black life story. But the psychological insights offered in those texts also have very special value, especially because the stories are from men and women who come from varied socioeconomic, historical, educational, religious, color, and work backgrounds.

The personal story is a helpful document about life at a given time because it tends to put flesh on the bones of a historical period that may be captured only incompletely by statistics and other summary data. What slave narrators, for example, say about their lives as slaves is worth hearing, even if their narratives evoke more questions about the inner lives of slaves than the stories ultimately answer. But think what our contemplations about slavery would be like if they were not informed by the personal ruminations of slaves themselves.

Still, recounting a life history isn't free of complexity. The autobiography, for example, cannot be expected to escape the critical analysis given to other art forms. That is why the careful reader wants to know the reason for the author's decision to tell his story: whether the author is seeking to set the record straight about some particular set of facts, whether the author's recall is being subjected to psychological or other duress, what the author may be deliberately or unconsciously including or excluding. In reading the personal stories of others, we should not be expected to suspend all our critical faculties.

I have always wanted to know what Malcolm X believed was his own version of the truth, even if I would then have trouble accepting it. By any measure, Malcolm was one of the important Black leaders of this country's Civil Rights movement in the 1960s and a major figure in one of the new African American religious movements of the twentieth century. The autobiographical explication of his relationship with his mentor, Elijah Muhammad, like the description of his parents and his early love of White women, had to be made by him. Even if, under later scrutiny by readers, the story would seem to spring holes, it still serves as Malcolm's version and no one else's. It is Malcolm's reality, which deserves serious consideration no matter what one's standards are for determining historical or psychological truth. But I still have questions about his story and would continue to have them even if the story had been related by a historian, anthropologist, sociologist, or other professional. It is obvious and accepted that even apparently objective professionals can be found guilty of grinding some distinctly personal axe. So storytelling is not without its problems.

One can hardly forget Erik Erikson's brilliant reminder, articulated in *Gandhi's Truth*, about the complexity of delineating clearly a particular individual's version of the truth. It was one thing to have Gandhi talk about his idea of nonviolence and quite another to have Erikson subject Gandhi's claims to concentrated psychological scrutiny. Gandhi's inner fears, once bared and examined, leave him looking more violent than one might at first have expected.

Sara Lawrence-Lightfoot has demonstrated, in her collection of stories titled *I've Known Rivers*, another genre for shedding light on the accomplishments of African Americans. In that format, Lawrence-Lightfoot is the medium through whom other actors talk about themselves. They relate the stories to her, and she takes the responsibility for structuring the tale and retelling it in her own words. One distinct advantage of this technique is that it avoids the wait until the subject decides to relate the story in autobiographical form. In addition, the intermediate medium may bring expertise and energy to the task that actually facilitate explication and understanding of complex individuals and their achievements.

Still, I can readily see that this form of telling stories has some apparent problems. The intermediary storyteller can easily approach the task with prejudice and then order, emphasize, or diminish events in the subject's life in a way that ultimately distorts the original version of the individual's story. There is, as far as I can tell, no way of correcting perfectly the lens through which an individual autobiographer sees the world or the hearing aid through which the storyteller first hears the facts from his subject. That is why there is a natural temptation to use witnesses to buttress certain crucial aspects of another individual's story, to add external support and weight to the idea that the story is in some way verifiable. Of course, the task is not to overdo it and then recount competing or multiple stories. But there is an unsuppressible urge to know what key bystanders, such as relatives and the spouse, think of an individual's version of reality. This third genre is what I call storytelling with extra precautions, although it is not clear whether this cautious form of storytelling is necessarily more accurate than other techniques. After all, does anyone seriously believe there is such a thing as an objective spouse?

James Comer's *Maggie's American Dream* and James McBride's *The Color of Water* are recent examples of another attempt at recounting the complete tale. Both of these authors tell at least part of their own personal story while relating what they have been told by their mothers. In each case the result is a mesmerizing collage of intersecting and interactional views of two different witnesses to a longitudinal family drama that really has no beginning or end. This fourth genre of telling the individual story certainly has its advantages. If nothing else, it is a shorthand way of getting at roots, at background, while a principal witness to the story is still around to give testimony. The work of these authors definitely makes it clear how truly difficult it is to reconstruct the life story when the major witnesses are all dead. Indeed, their contributions suggest to me that we ought to find some name other than *biography* to describe the process of storytelling from textual data, from reconstructed artifacts that lack the living human voice.

It is my hope that the methodological weaknesses of each genre of storytelling can be at least outweighed, if not completely overcome, by the achievement of having a story delineated in enough detail to fill the void created by the story's nonexistence. In other words, when the story's telling is over, we ought to feel that we are better off for having heard the story and for having enhanced our knowledge of the story's subject. This is a case where a half loaf is surely better than nothing at all.

It is that feeling of discontent about a missing story that has so drawn me to recount the life of Chester Pierce, an African American psychiatrist who has had a profound effect on American psychiatry and on the thinking of African American psychiatrists and professionals from other mental health disciplines, particularly during the past two decades. Although he has authored substantive scholarship on the task of coping with extreme environments, such as the South Pole, Chester Pierce is probably best known among psychiatrists and other mental health professionals for his theories about how Blacks cope with racist behavior in the United States.

I first met Pierce around 1976 when he was giving a lecture at the Albert Einstein College of Medicine. He sat in a chair and talked extemporaneously for almost an hour, in an exquisitely ordered fashion that brought to mind the lectures I had so often experienced during my stay in Europe. He obviously followed the outline he had made in his mind, and his performance prompted one of my Einstein teachers to remark to me that Pierce had done what was expected of distinguished Harvard professors. Obviously, he had performed brilliantly. He had held his audience.

Pierce's own accomplishments are singularly striking, especially when viewed in their historical context. He was born in 1927; by 1952, he was a graduate of the Harvard Medical School, having already taken his undergraduate degree at Harvard College. He went on to become president of the American Board of Psychiatry and Neurology in 1978 and president of the American Orthopsychiatric Association in 1983, and he was appointed during his career to the editorial boards of 22 publications and elected to the world-famous Institute of Medicine at the National Academy of Sciences in 1971. In 1969, he was the founding national chair of the Black Psychiatrists of America, and in 1988 the National Medical Association named an annual research seminar after him. By any measure, Pierce has emerged as one of the true lights in twentieth-century American psychiatry, one of the few individuals with substantive standing in both the Black and White mental health communities.

I do not believe there is another American psychiatrist whose theoretical musings about racism are more commonly used in the everyday workplace of mental health clinicians. It is Pierce who has caused so many of us to talk about the constant microtraumas that the racially oppressed individual must endure, of racism as an environmental pollutant, of the state of defensive thinking that so characterizes the oppressed, and of the offensive mechanisms employed by the racist oppressor.

A number of questions naturally emerge when one thinks about Chester Pierce. How has he managed to pull together in his professional thinking so many disparate themes? How, for example, are extreme environments linked to questions of racism? But on a more personal level, who is this man who has managed to graduate twice from Harvard? What is his wife like, and how has he raised his children? How has he personally coped with the microtraumas and macrotraumas of everyday racist actions? What are his views on religion, and for what particular accomplishment would he like to be remembered? I do not believe that a recitation of Pierce's academic writings would really tell very much about the man. Discussing his life story and excluding his profound thinking in the psychiatric arena would be equally unsatisfactory. I wish to meld together the man and his work and emerge with a cohesive and coherent story about the person everybody likes to call Chet.

I have repeatedly turned over in my mind the question of why I wanted to tell his story and not someone else's. Certainly, one aspect of the answer has to do with the complicated reasons we all choose our heroes. But another part of the answer relates to the inherent nature of telling other people's stories—and leads me to the conclusion that I want to do more than tell Chet Pierce's story. In recognizing that, I've come to understand my lack of satisfaction with using any of the other techniques I've just described to talk about Chet. They do not allow me to get into Chet's story, to delve below the words.

It finally dawned on me that I wanted the chance to carry on a sort of argumentative dialogue with him. I recognize that I am seduced by the task of having to hold his feet to the fire, so to speak. For a long time I have contemplated having the opportunity to urge Chet to clarify his positions; and I have so earnestly wanted to explore his logic and question him about whatever contradictions might be found in his thinking. In a way, I have carried out this dialogue so consistently in my mind over the years with no other intellectual in American psychiatry. This has, of course, persuaded me that Chet's story ultimately has something to do with helping me better conceptualize my own.

After all is said and done, I cannot help noting that in stark Levinsonian terms, that is to say, in the framework so artfully constructed by Daniel Levinson and his colleagues in *The Seasons of a Man's Life*, I am entering the culmination of middle adulthood and struggling to complete my age-fifty transitional period. Chet, having been born in 1927, is well into late adulthood and obviously contemplating the age-seventy transition. He must therefore have something to teach me about modification of my own life structure, and I want to discuss it with him. So yes, it's evident that I never wanted just to tell Chet's story; I wanted to work his story out, to measure it, to try it on, to figure out which parts are good for me and for other Blacks so earnestly seeking heroes.

Continuing My Dialogue With Chester Pierce

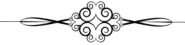

INTRODUCTION TO THE REVISED EDITION

Chester Pierce called me his "biographer," and sometimes he used the term in introducing me to others. He and I both laughed on occasion when he said it. However, composing the narrative of his life from our exchanges gradually became more important than I had imagined it would be. I found myself in a sustained relationship that lasted until a short time before his death. That is when he became more introspective, and we talked less frequently. I concluded that he wished to be left to contemplate quietly the outcome of his illness. Once the book was finished, and until his withdrawal, we spoke regularly by telephone. He had a long life. Born in 1927 in Glen Cove, New York, he retired at age 70 from his professorship at the Harvard Medical School and the Harvard Graduate School of Education. He died on September 23, 2016, at 89.

I believe Pierce and I first met when he came to deliver a lecture at New York's Lincoln Hospital around 1976. My training director had arranged for Pierce and me to chat. The encounter was a significant event in my life and the beginning of an excursion with an extraordinary man.

Our telephone discussions, after publication of *Race and Excellence* and commencement of Pierce's retirement, were wide-ranging. They swung from the personal to considerations of regional, national, and international issues. He was always interested in family matters, both his and mine. He dwelled often on the good fortune that he had experienced. There was no looking back with regret or disgust. He had no time to chat negatively about individuals who had not been friendly toward him. In that spirit, he often guided the conversation to questions of administrative import related to my activities at work. He had been an academic for many years. This allowed him to get quickly to the crux of problems. He understood transactions and context, the connection of personality structure and power dynamics, and the influence of discrimination of all sorts on systemic structures.

Background

In talking about *Race and Excellence*, I often emphasize that I was the sole narrator in the project. I formulated the story of the interactions between Chester Pierce and me. The accounts and his voice came through my pen, although I did my best to preserve the authenticity of what he recounted. The promise to be accurate was important. I have always had profound respect for him as mentor, colleague, and friend. He welcomed me as a participant in his civil rights and human rights struggles. We constantly discussed the different geographies in which we operated. I spent extensive time in Barbados between 1980 and 2020 carrying out scholarly projects. I enjoyed constructing life stories of individuals from that island. I saw the people I met there as witnesses to the act of living life in their communities, in their times, in a postcolonial context. (Chester Pierce would be interested to know that a few days ago, Barbados became a democratic republic with a Barbadian president. The ties to Great Britain and its queen have been cut.) Sometimes, we moved in and out of each other's lives as the years went by. I used a similar approach in my discussions with Chester Pierce, although I was more systematic in talking to him regularly in his Harvard University office for a couple of years. He was in his late sixties at the time, as I remember interviewing him about his impending retirement at age 70.

After years of doing biographical and autobiographical work, I acknowledge my love and respect for the human voice. I have written about narrative for at least the past 25 years. After the 1998 publication of *Race and Excellence*, I wrote a 2005 family memoir (*I'm Your Father, Boy*) that was set in Barbados, so influenced by the historical context of British colonialism. In 2010, I published *Ye Shall Dream* on the life of a deeply religious modern prophet who founded a faith group new to Barbados. These forms of narrative scholarship evolved from courses I taught in African American studies at Yale University. One course focused on Black autobiographies from different social, professional, and psychological perspectives. We discussed slave narratives and stories from pastors, politicians, musicians, dancers, actors, and others. The second course addressed biographical storytelling among Caribbean authors. I melded the themes I cultivated in those two sets of curricula with principles and attitudes acquired in the practice of social and community psychiatry. In addition, I borrowed heavily from anthropological discourse in developing my approach to narrative employed in psychiatry.

In looking at storytelling techniques used by writers, it is evident that authors make use of a variety of aesthetic approaches and structures. Consider briefly, as examples, just three books in the past 25 years from psychiatrists who used narrative as a fundamental structural and communicative platform: *City of One: A Memoir* by Francine Cournos (Norton, 1999); *Women in Psychiatry: Personal Perspectives*, edited by D.M. Norris, G. Jayaram, and A.B. Primm (American Psychiatric Publishing, 2012); and *The Soul of Care: The Moral Education of a Husband and a Doctor* by Arthur Kleinman (Viking, 2019). Cournos issued a fascinating and personal story of her life, characterized by the early loss of both parents and her struggle to adjust and adapt psychologically and socially. It is a compelling example of the classic case history. *Women in Psychiatry* is an edited collection of stories from female psychiatrists. The thematic emphasis is on the female voice, cultivated in a single profession, although varying in cultural perspective. Kleinman, a psychiatrist-anthropologist, reported on his experience of caring for his wife, who progressively deteriorated functionally and cognitively at the hands of dementia. It is a thoughtful narrative focused on the intricacies of caring for a human being; the horror of witnessing, up close, the systematic deterioration of a loved one; and the absence of compassion in modern medicine. The three books are important and present themes that demand reflection from members of our discipline. *Race and Excellence* is conceptually different from the texts I have just mentioned. It also contrasts appreciably with my later work in terms of both structure and content. It extended my early thinking about narrative in terms of geography, culture, politics, and social relations. It encompasses two intertwined single lives, more than one unique culture, and more than a single theme. *Race and Excellence* relies on both biographical and self-portraiture approaches.

Writing about Chester Pierce, I wanted to focus on his individuality. One reader of an early draft of the book wanted me to highlight context more and to dwell on my interpretation of his life. However, I wanted the meaning to emerge from his voice and our interactive discourse. I wished to have him discuss his struggles and the techniques he employed to cope with the displeasures. Then, I would react. I concentrated on capturing his accounts and exploring his conceptualizations of home, work, and leisure; on hearing about who and what he wanted to become, about what blocked or facilitated his dreams. I was interested in his quest to put his stamp on different aspects of public policy. I took pleasure in recounting what he said about understanding the major landscapes he occupied, his relationship with God, the regrets in the life he lived. I could then examine his ideas from different angles. I did my best to focus the light on two Black men, professors of psychiatry, from geographies miles apart, just talking.

Contextualizing the New Edition

It is now more than two decades since the original version of *Race and Excellence* was published in 1998. The turn into the twenty-first century has been, at least to me, surprisingly eventful, especially in the past few years. That is when events started to push relaxing, mundane matters to the side. Professor Hazel Carby, in a January 2021 essay ("The Limits of Caste," *London Review of Books*) talked of the "material and symbolic anxieties of the present" that began around 2016 with the change in the presidency of the United States. Then, "a sense of emergency, of imminent threat" became palpable. Carby described the following 4 years as characterized by "increasing authoritarianism and the rampant spread of White supremacist hatred and violence."

However, the new Republican president's rhetoric and actions from 2016 to 2020, while certainly important, did not cause all of the turmoil. We also had the ongoing problem of race relations melded with new discussions of what caste meant. Isabel Wilkerson fueled some of those conversations with publication of her text *Caste: The Origins of Our Discontents* (Random House, 2020). The question followed: How can we make things better between dominant group members and those lacking fiscal resources and human dignity, the ones at the bottom of the caste ladder? Even the American Psychiatric Association, my main professional group, held meetings over months seeking to contend with the caustic interactions of race and organizational making of policy. I have been stunned, too, by the open political strife and violence in the countries I know best. It seems widespread, this mocking of others on the basis of ethnicity, skin color, social standing, and impoverished socioeconomic resources. There are also the powerful effects of the coronavirus pandemic on the unfolding of this new century. It taught us about our inherent powerlessness in the face of certain natural events and the need to depend on each other at times when selfishness and competition seem embarrassingly useless and irrelevant.

The Reprinted Text

I believe that happenings of the past few years have partly influenced the decision to reprint *Race and Excellence*. Chester Pierce's work has illuminated the connection between racial/ethnic discrimination and much of what has been taking place around us. Even recent events, such as the upheaval in Afghanistan and the devastating effects of the earthquake in Haiti, have a connection to the theorizing of Pierce. Both geographic spaces are remarkably obvious extreme environments. In both contexts, physical and mental health are at risk because of the aggravated caste systems operating in the two cultures. The dialogues between Pierce and me that characterize *Race and Excellence* highlight the linkages between psychiatry and richly racialized national and international cultures. The dialogues have also contributed to increased recognition of Chester Pierce's contributions to American psychiatry and to common cultural discourse about matters of race and justice. Certainly, his concept of mundane microaggressions as a significant manifestation of discrimination is now in common use. Similarly, we understand better how oppression is manifest in efforts to control another's space, time, and energy.

The appearance of the new text may coincide with a resurgence of interest in and endowment of the American Psychiatric Association's Chester M. Pierce Human Rights Award. The award recognizes the extraordinary efforts of individuals and organizations and sheds light on their efforts to promote the human rights of populations with mental health needs. It was originally established in 1990 to raise awareness of human rights abuses but was renamed in 2017 to honor Dr. Pierce. It highlights his dedication as an innovative researcher on individuals living in extreme environments; his advocacy against stigma, discrimination, and disparities in health; and his strong commitment to the concept of global mental health.

Constructing a new introduction for this edition of *Race and Excellence* helps me to see the influence of Pierce on my own work. At the time I decided to write about his life, I was interested in the connection between life stories and the Black community in the United States, as well as the place of Blacks in organizations such as universities. I thought that focusing on him was, to some extent, opening a window onto Black life and culture. The melding of his biography with certain features of my own story was a unique way, I thought, of testing certain ideas about Black life cross-nationally. Those interests of 20 years ago remain. However, they are now linked to other sociocultural experiences, such as the effects of climate change, the raucous presence of the coronavirus, and the persistent problems provoked by ethnicity and class in America and elsewhere.

Imagining a Continuing Dialogue

Chester Pierce and I should be discussing current matters now, periodically, say, once a month. I would mention how friends were coping in Barbados or France. He would theorize more broadly about how the Turks were doing and why the Chinese were strategically making their moves to outfox the Western politicians. Chet, which was my term of endearment for him, would point out that the COVID-19 pandemic, with its isolation and death, provoked reactive responses of institutions to its dominance. He would perhaps suggest that the coronavirus has taught us anew about reordering our social and economic priorities. It has forced us to think about the meaning of mundane rituals and values we have long taken for granted.

I have wondered what he would think of my being troubled by the renewed reliance on the public lie and the enhanced emphasis on disinformation all around us. I am not accustomed to this use of mendacity for all to see. I am familiar with the hesitant use of deceit and sleight of hand in private discourse, under wraps, so to speak. However, I am not friends with the technique of publicly promoting demonstrably false concepts such as the notion that the coronavirus is easily controlled and a mere passing annoyance. I also mention here the problem of *monster stories*. I borrow the term from Gwen Adshead, a British psychiatrist-friend of mine who worries about its currency and ubiquity. She referred to these stories in her work on serious crimes committed by people living with severe mental illness. Some observers paint these individuals as concentrated villains, evil and destructive. The person lacks even a scintilla of redeeming possibility, and the portrait is intended to frighten the community. It is sad when one uses the monster story to demean the other and to gain advantage over the individual who is portrayed as almost less than human. Monster portraits are especially obnoxious when linked with fake news about an individual. Chester Pierce was concerned about these techniques and recognized their use at times against minority groups. I was familiar with their use against migrants, especially when I heard tales about Caribbean friends trying to make a new life in London or New York. I also saw the phenomenon up close when serving as a soldier in Vietnam. Then, the image of the Vietnamese as monsters was at the core of American rhetoric.

I would tell Chet about having attended a 2021 reception in Birmingham, one of the United Kingdom's most diverse cities. I had the good fortune to meet a member of the worldwide Quaker movement. We discussed his religious group's tenets and basic rituals. Then he summarized his belief that humanity is now at a "point of great turning." He saw the possibilities of cooperatively confronting the major challenges of climate change; race-based, gender-based, and class-based injustice; general inequality; and violence. He maintained that his views were undergirded by the biblical text from Micah 6:8: "He has shown you, O man, what is good. And what does the Lord require of you but to act justly, to love mercy, and to walk humbly with your God?"

Chet and I could easily emphasize the religious dimension of my new friend's ideas. However, it seemed to me that one could see religion as representing a thin patina on notions of living. I am thinking here of Greg Epstein, the humanist chaplain at Harvard University, and his provocative text, *Good Without God* (William Morrow, 2009). The point is that one can accomplish good in life by seeking constructive purpose, treating others with compassion, and building community. Similarly, my British friend saw the problems around him as existing across all the continents, irrespective of citizens' religious beliefs. He offered an open, collaborative approach to the solutions that, in his view, demanded cooperation from each of us. Similarly, Chet talked about the principles by which we could live, without framing things in a religious context. He was preoccupied with the implementation of justice in multiple domains. Furthermore, those who knew him spoke easily of his humility and remarkable generosity. He and I focused, from time to time, on his churchgoing, and he encouraged my research on Black church rituals and the role of the Black church as a healing community. I also had the impression that his spiritual life was private and rarely advertised. Nevertheless, he had little patience for religious ideas that divided people from their neighbors, promoted our vanity, increased competition, and visibly left one group or another at the bottom of the caste ladder. I recognized that the failings of organized religion did not stop him from appreciating the inherent therapeutic value of faith-based communities.

Reflecting on these points, I gradually understood that Chet visualized greater breadth in the portrait of the world around him than I appreciated at first. He liked the combination of narratives from different cultures, products of dialogue between him and others sometimes, and related to others he was observing. He enjoyed the focus on individuals' reactions to experiences and events in their lives. The contextual background was the cultural fabric weaved around people. On an international scale, powerful forces influence the formation of our backgrounds. Some examples are racialized and class-based political disputes, identity politics that defy easy resolution, and pervasive feelings of individual disenchantment. There is also the search for a sense of human dignity and personal worth and uncertainty about the future in terms of health and security. The pandemic has turned those catalysts upside down and produced extensive dislocation in the general culture. Chet did not know of this latest plague, but he was ahead of most of us because of his interest in extreme environments and the challenge to control climate's independence.

Readers and the Text

I hope that, regardless of one's vantage point, the interactive dialogue between Chester Pierce and me appeals to readers and leads to reflection about our conversations. We discuss our life experiences and engage in quiet meaning-making. Our exchanges may require some concentration and a commitment to the adventure of reading about our lives that unfolds in contrasting times and places. The two lives have some similarities and intriguing differences. There is, too, the privilege of seeing how we have confronted Eriksonian events in our lives and then agreed to recount our experiences through the power of stories. Borrowing language from Shoshana Felman and Dori Laub in their popular text, *Testimony* (Routledge, 1992), the life stories I narrate "cover a whole spectrum of concerns, issues, works, and media of transmission, moving from the literary to the visual, from the artistic to the autobiographical…to the historical" (p. XV). Stories always have the potential to serve as models for contemplation of reactions to turmoil and dislocation. They also serve well as a culture-based way of framing future developments in public policy. People's life stories and experiences chart a course for political and legislative decision-making about race and health, race and education, race and criminal justice. Readers of *Race and Excellence* will confront the written experiences of others and also think about whether the accounts make sense in their imagination. Readers will think about their own lives and whether the stories usefully fit them or are just temporary fantastical flights away from their realities.

A colleague recently spoke to me of an early speech given by Chet to a group of educators that was published in 1972 under the title of "Becoming Planetary Citizens" (*Childhood Education* 49:58-63, 1972). In the piece, Chet tackled the problem of preparing young students for the twenty-first century, to live in a world as planetary citizens. He envisaged their being mindful of interacting with others beyond national geographic boundaries and being acutely aware of the need to be collaborative rather than simply competitive. That would, he thought, require a higher level of general knowledge about the world and its nations. This would produce more supergeneralists seeking the status of planetary citizenship. He argued it would augment the pursuit of hope in the place of selfish and destructive competition. With this objective in mind, Chet saw the need for educators to focus on such matters as conflict resolution, decision-making, the international spread of infectious diseases, and the effects of technology on life everywhere.

The characteristic features of this speech, published 50 years ago, were based on thinking broadly about the dignity of individuals. One sees in it the imperative of understanding how local action produces repercussions across the globe. Chet argued in this article that racism is the pernicious impediment to achieving the desired objective of collaborative citizenship. Racism is a pollutant that interferes with interactive and productive fellowship. Seeing people in your neighborhood as the other, that individual you do not know and whom you fear and see as different and inferior, automatically makes it harder to establish global interactions that are mutually beneficial. That is why Chet talked repeatedly of seeing travel as a way of exploring mutual humanity. I believe, too, that there is a connection between these futuristic, inter-nation ideas of Chet and the hope that we will eventually deal with each other nonviolently.

Unfinished Business

I confess that I have had some misgivings about unfinished business with Chet. There are two matters that I have turned over in my mind on repeated occasions. The first concerns his tenacious and repetitive conclusion that a sense of belonging at Harvard always eluded him. This was perhaps the most problematic claim that emerged in our discussions. I took note of facts and incidents that seemed to establish his grounding at Harvard. He had obtained his bachelor's degree there, played on its varsity football team, attended its medical school, held a professorial appointment in the School of Education and the Medical School for many years. He and I had walked around Cambridge, dined at the small city's numerous ethnic restaurants, and encountered other faculty members in the street who greeted him deferentially. He had taken me to the Harvard Faculty Club, where the rituals and architecture combine to make its users feel they have certainly arrived, even if they are uncomfortable in its precincts. He had also told me about the portrait of him that Harvard had commissioned, to be hung within some university space.

Surrounded by such evidence, I found it hard to grasp the legitimacy of his assertion. It felt like the statement of a military strategist who has spent years planning the effort to take a city only to state, after winning the war and taking up residence in the land he has conquered, that he could never enjoy living there. Chet was interred without our having returned to this conversation. We also did not review my latest book, *Belonging, Therapeutic Landscapes, and Networks* (Routledge, 2018), in which I articulated my hesitancy in making claims about belonging at Yale, after teaching there for almost 40 years. In the interim, I had read the important essay-letter "To Sit at the Welcome Table" by Harvard's former president, Drew Faust (*Harvard Magazine*, July 2014). Faust documented Harvard's efforts over centuries to make minority group members feel tolerated and barely welcome at the university. She pointed out the changes wrought in recent years to change that aspect of Harvard. She referred to the inspiration in Langston Hughes' poem "I, Too," and she conjured up the image of Harvard as a welcome table. She promised sustained renewal of the efforts to guarantee everyone at Harvard an honored seat at the table. It is of considerable interest, too, that Yale and other universities have recently been discussing publicly their considerable participation in the institution of slavery. Chet would have had much comment to make about this happening, had he lived to witness it.

The writings of scholars at these distinguished institutions often ring with sincerity of purpose and commitment. It is easy to believe them. On the other hand, those a little lower on the totem pole of university administration can make decisions that convey a surprising lack of compassion and concern for their charges' dignity. I was concerned about the virulence of competition and emphasis on self-interest at Yale. I understood that the idea of planetary citizenship, fueled by collaboration and mutual respect within a community of individuals with common interests, was not popular in the spaces I frequented. Having said that, it is a pleasure to note that changes have been made, and progress is in the air. The national conversation about race matters has left its mark in the ivory tower of academia.

The second piece of unfinished business that I have pondered from time to time in connection with Chester Pierce has been the subject of self-exile. Black people have been energetic participants in the phenomenon of geographic migration over many generations. Scholars have discussed, for example, the early- and mid-twentieth-century movement of Southern Blacks in the United States to cities in the North and West. Similar consideration has been given to Caribbean Blacks and their relocation to the United Kingdom and the United States during the 1950s and 1960s. The 2021 reissue of William Gardner Smith's *The Stone Face* by the *New York Review of Books* has rekindled interest in the self-exile of Black artists and other intellectuals from the United States to France in the twentieth century. It is of some note, too, that one of the critics of my scholarship once labeled me a Caribbean exile. I have always assumed that the label conveyed some unexplained meaning about my having settled in North America from Barbados and later studying medicine in France. In his scholarly introduction to the new edition of *The Stone Face*, Adam Shatz focused on the exile of people such as Richard Wright, James Baldwin, the cartoonist Ollie Harrington, William Gardner Smith, Josephine Baker, and Sidney Bechet. Shatz commented that Paris offered to these individuals a refuge from segregation and discrimination and opened a more normal everyday life to them. Part of the mundane normalcy included opportunities to interact with everybody, to enjoy acceptance by shopkeepers and police officials, and to cultivate a strong ethnic and personal identity.

Shatz was quick to point out that this common exile to France, which occurred between the 1920s and the American Civil Rights years, had its own dangers. American Blacks' welcome by French authorities did not mean that France had no caste-based discrimination in operation. Indeed, France was shown to operate a caste ladder effectively, with Algerians and Black Africans on the bottom. The other problem was that leaving the United States behind did not efface the American problem. All it possibly meant was that those who departed U. S. shores relinquished civil rights efforts to those who remained at home. The issue became a serious difficulty, in terms of philosophy, policy, and ethics, for the group of exiles. That is why several of them returned home to participate in the civil rights activities and clear their names of any suspicion that they had abandoned the struggle to others.

I did not directly discuss the self-exile question with Chet. Nevertheless, we did talk about whether participation in resolving these moral dilemmas was mandatory. As a general principle, he affirmed the obligation to give something back to the society in which one was reared. He stated that doctors, because they had received so much in terms of esteem, prestige, and salary, should contribute some of their time, energy, and money to those who were less fortunate. He lived by example in these matters. So, in his terms, he put a brick regularly toward construction of civil rights and human rights efforts. He did so without fanfare. The unwelcome noise distracted him.

He often reminded me that evaluating the reasons others give for their decisions assumed that the critics had complete and accurate knowledge of what drove the actions of those under scrutiny. Chet believed that those evaluations were often wrong. So he affirmed his commitment to struggling against the oppression of Blacks, both at home and abroad. He defined the struggle in international terms, or in global terms, as is now the preferred terminology. We never discussed the matter of searching for Zion outside the United States. However, I did not believe that he saw some other country as the proverbial land of milk and honey, at least as far as race relations were concerned. In *Search for Zion* (Atlantic Press, 2013), Emily Raboteau, for example, takes the reader around the globe and returns to the possibility that home is within oneself. Certainly, some of the Paris self-exiles reached the same conclusion and found home back in the United States or in some other country. A colleague did ask me whether Chet's extensive traveling to fulfill his scholarly commitments may have represented a form of respite or self-imposed distancing from the stress of the unceasing struggle against injustice. On reflection, I must accept the possibility of such a hypothesis. These days, it comes under the heading of self-care. I can confirm that Chet was very concerned about the heavy price paid by the Black body and mind in daily racialized living.

Adam Shatz points to an important finding in the work of William Gardner Smith: the rootlessness that often accompanies self-exile. I observed how Chet participated vigorously in civil rights work at home. I concluded easily that such activity, coupled with his clinical and intellectual efforts in medicine, provided a solid identity base for him. This was reinforced by his family and marriage ties. What may one make of his stated lack of belonging at Harvard, an institution that provided him so much pleasure and honor? Is this a form of rootlessness that comes from the chronic pain inflicted in the struggle on behalf of the oppressed? I ask because I know that the small incremental successes achieved in the years-long civil rights struggles can be hard to take. Chet mentioned that idea to me on several occasions in his neurophysiology theorizing about the stress on those in the struggle. The grand victory is the rare conclusion, and it is shared by only a few. I wish I had been able to explore this matter in greater depth with Chet. Such thoughts do keep him alive.

Ezra E.H. Griffith, M.D.
December 2021

1

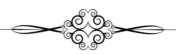

The Beginnings and Glen Cove

The telephone message said that I should meet him in front of the Greek columns of the Harvard Coop, and he was there on time, sitting with his arms folded while he intently followed the activities of passersby. It was not surprising to me that he was early, of course, because I knew he took commitments seriously, especially when they were made to brothers or sisters in the struggle. So I never doubted he would be there. As he recognized me, he stood up and shook my hand warmly, while I took in his full height of 6 feet 4 inches. Then we strolled over to a German restaurant in Harvard Square, ate lunch, and chatted about the project that was going to occupy us for a number of months.

It was a good beginning. Chester Middlebrook Pierce, professor of education, psychiatry, and public health at Harvard University, was about to tell me the story of his life and work. I was pleased by his decision, since his reputation alone had given me the sense that his story would be captivating. Furthermore, I simply could not imagine a more significant intellectual privilege than having the opportunity to talk to him at length about how he had built his career, what had motivated his interests, and why certain subjects had so captured his fancy. But I was also taken by his decision to tell his story through my pen. After all, it must require enormous trust to cede the recounting of your life story to someone else, especially to a foreign-born "outsider." Although we had a good deal in common professionally, Chet was an African American and I had grown up in Barbados, truly a world apart. But our careers and our shared interest in not only the history but the future of Black people in this country had brought us together for this project.

I was conscious that it had been decades since I was first with Chet in a similarly private context. I was still in specialty training at that time. He had been invited to give a lecture at the hospital where I was doing my residency, and the director of training thought I should have the opportunity to interact privately with this world-renowned professor. Chester Pierce talked that day about how to conceptualize the development of a career. He insisted that one ought to think dynamically about setting up a curriculum vitae. He counseled that toward the end of every academic year, individuals should try to think dispassionately about what they had accomplished, assessing the articles published, speeches made, courses taught, and service provided to committees. In that way, one could actually plot the course of any career movement over a 5-year period. It was his view that such objective assessment would also afford the opportunity for modifying one's course in midstream and for determining whether a particular direction was really the one that provided personal satisfaction.

At the time, he also advocated strongly that Blacks participate vigorously in White-dominated professional organizations and that Blacks learn what true excellence was, regardless of its source. Several years later, I began to appreciate fully that there were other Black psychiatrists who argued that Black professionals like themselves should interact only with organizations dominated by Blacks. So Chet's critical thinking had an important political dimension to it. Of course, what I didn't know at that first meeting with him was that certain parts of this practical philosophy had been generated by his father, who had spent a lifetime observing Whites in their own habitat and distilling what he thought he needed in order to provide well for himself and his family. The senior Samuel Pierce clearly did not have a narrow vision of his sons wielding power only in Black-dominated institutions. For him, the entire world was potentially their stage.

At the Harvard Square lunch, I took note of several characteristics as I observed Chester Pierce. For instance, I noted that he ordered a lot to eat; then I realized that he really had a big frame to feed, although he weighed only about 220 pounds. But a most striking feature was his uncommon mannerliness, a trait I would learn later had to have come from the combined influence of his stylish father and his rule-bound mother. Both parents would have fostered a certain deportment in their children because they recognized manners as an obvious sign of good breeding. The unusual civility would also have been reinforced later during Chester Pierce's undergraduate years as a resident in Harvard

College's Lowell House, where Master Elliott Perkins held sway and invited students to High Table in their formal dinner jackets.

Chet's reference to Harvard reminded me that I, too, was a product of Lowell House, although a full 15 years after he was there. In talking with him, I became aware of my own diminished enthusiasm about my Lowell House years and I recognized that he espoused a stricter attitude than I toward manners and customs that I had come to associate with British colonialism, a result of my own upbringing in the West Indies. For example, Chet still believed men ought to stand up when women entered a room. He was also uncomfortable eating dinner without wearing a jacket and tie, an obvious holdover from the Lowell House days, when dining without a cravat of some sort was an immutable prohibition. (It wasn't lost on me that I was wearing an open-necked shirt while lunching with this African American gentleman.) Chet earnestly loved these matters of personal elegance and firmly believed that doctors should be gentlemen.

Over lunch, we mused about my ideas regarding the telling of stories, and I tried to explain how and why I had decided that his story was an important one to recount. We discussed the course I had developed at Yale on the study of Black autobiographies and my growing conviction that the examination of Black lives was an important window on what was happening in the Black community, on the ideas being developed there, and on the culture that Blacks were constantly fashioning and refashioning. We discussed how important it was for our Black heroes to be better understood, a difficult task if one examined only an individual's writings or other professional productions. We eventually strolled back to his office located on the third floor of a quaint building on Appian Way, just off Harvard Square. For some reason, I wasn't expecting the furnishings of his professorial den to be so spare. But I was also instantly taken by the quiet isolation of the office and its obvious relationship to scholarly productivity. We quickly settled in and then launched into the task at hand.

Chester Pierce was born in 1927 in Glen Cove, New York, a small Long Island community with a population then of 8,000, about 800 of whom were Black. It was a relatively rural area, within 25 miles of New York City, made up of a village, houses, some farms, and giant estates owned by very rich people. There was solid racial friendliness in Glen Cove at that time and generally good neighborliness, so young Chester led a life with minimal—but still some—racial stress.

Chet was the second of three children born to Samuel Pierce and Hettie Armstrong, a couple who had married in 1909 in the small town of Hertford, North Carolina. Samuel was about 23 years old at the time they married, and Hettie was 16. It is not clear what Samuel Pierce was doing courting a small-town North Carolinian, and he talked very little of those bygone days to his children. But it seems he met Hettie when he took a trip to Hertford to visit a friend. Samuel was born in Portsmouth, Virginia, in the year 1884. He was just a toddler when his father died, and he was raised by his mother, Chinnie Poyner. His father's early passing may have been the reason Samuel sought work so soon. As a child, he worked as a riveter in the Portsmouth Naval Shipyard; and he learned how to cut hair during the time he hung around barbershops sweeping up. Chet knew no more about Samuel's personal life in Virginia. For instance, he had no idea whether his father's forebears were slaves or not.

At about age 12, Samuel went to New York City by himself. He took a room in Harlem and worked at the Plaza Hotel, shining shoes and caring for the horses of the hotel's guests. Very soon he met a benefactor who helped him find work at a country club on the North Shore of Long Island. There, he grew from adolescence into manhood, becoming a naturally muscular, dark-skinned adult of medium height and weighing about 150 pounds. Samuel Pierce worked at the same country club until he died in 1943. He ran the locker room and also developed a private business on the side, barbering, shining club members' shoes, and cleaning and pressing their clothes. In addition, he tended bar and served food at members' private parties; he even accompanied some families on excursions in their private railroad cars. On those occasions, he was included in the families' activities, such as football games and other contexts reserved for those who were obviously advantaged.

Hettie Armstrong's background emerges more clearly in Chester Pierce's recollections. She grew up in Hertford and was quite familiar with racial issues of the time, sometimes talking about a brother who had to leave town because of a fight with a White man. Hettie had an interesting heritage. Her father was half Scottish and half Iroquois, and her mother was a mixture of Black, White, and Cherokee. She had no slaves among her familial antecedents. Hettie herself was a tall and buxom woman, light-skinned, and had long black hair reaching well down her back.

I have thought often of how much I know about my own parents' background. I can piece together substantially more about my father than I can about my mother, and I think I have been influenced by memories of my paternal grandfather. I still have intact a mental snapshot of my father's mother after her return from Europe, sitting on a large steamer trunk. In contrast, my mother's parents died working on the

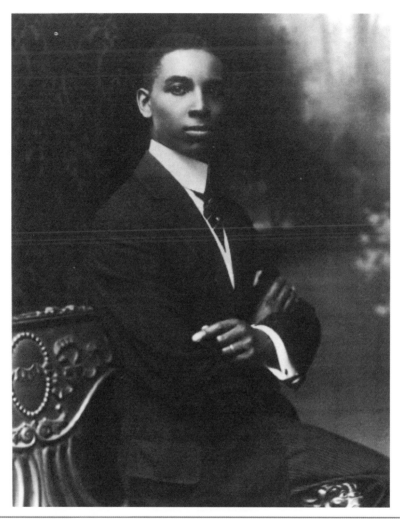

Samuel Pierce Sr., circa 1912.

Panama Canal, and she could not remember them. She was raised by a very strict aunt, whom I knew well but who never seemed to connect my mother to her Panama history. My father had several brothers and sisters whom I met over the years and who seemed to have substantially more presence in my early life than any of my mother's family.

For 13 years, Hettie tried unsuccessfully to become pregnant. Then she met a Spanish doctor who helped her improve her fertility. Her first child, Samuel (Junior), was born in 1922; 5 years later saw the arrival of 10.5-pound Chester; and in 1929, Burton saw the light of day. Hettie told Chet he was born with his skin all shriveled up and that she felt a lot of

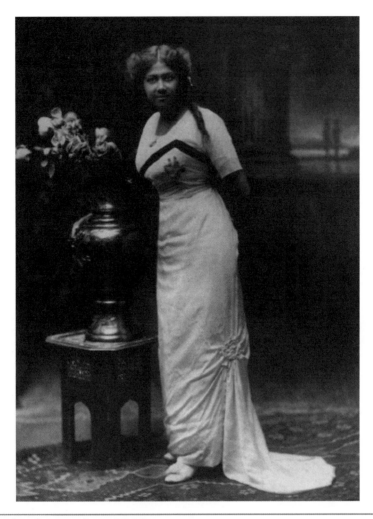

Hettie Pierce, circa 1912.

sympathy for him. Whether this sympathy was also evoked by his coming well past his due date or by the likelihood that his size might have made the delivery somewhat difficult is not clear.

Three male children turned the household into a "spirited and boy-oriented" place. Chet recalls how even distant relatives indulged the male offspring, a philosophy supported readily by his mother and an older female cousin who lived with the Pierce family. Although the boys had chores such as cutting the grass, those tasks seemed to follow an irregular pattern. Furthermore, the aunts continued the indulgence well into Chet's adulthood. He tells the story of his own wife preparing

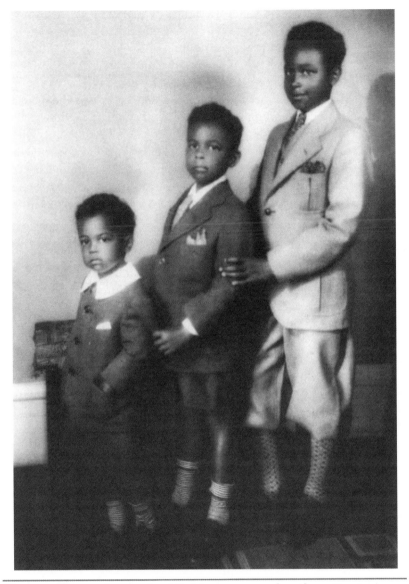

Chester Pierce *(center)* with his younger brother, Burton, and older brother, Samuel, circa 1933.

two eggs for him in the presence of his aunts. They remonstrated, telling his wife that she should have prepared half a dozen eggs for her spouse! Chet clearly enjoyed the indulgence and attention of females. It is a theme that recurs throughout his life: persistent yet subtle enough to be readily missed.

Young Chet attended Central Primary School in Glen Cove, and he did well. His performance was impressive enough that he was allowed to skip the seventh grade. This academic brilliance was reinforced by success in other arenas. When he was about 8 years old, he and some other children were playing hide-and-seek. By accident, Chet's younger brother fell into a well. An adult neighbor had witnessed the incident, but she remained standing on her porch, screaming pointlessly. Chet didn't hesitate; he quickly lowered a chain to his brother and, with a friend's help, pulled up young Burton. Chet emerged as a hero, which he concedes helped his uncertain self-esteem. An obese child, Chet was self-conscious about his size and felt he was not as good-looking as his brothers. His mother apparently remained sensitive to this family dynamic and did her best to protect him from the repeated comments of outsiders who were quick to applaud the handsome appearance of Chet's siblings.

At age 10, Chet went off to Camp Atwater, a Massachusetts summer spot where many privileged Blacks sent their children for the long annual vacation break. His older brother had been there, but it was Chet's first experience in a predominantly Black setting, apart from the African Methodist Episcopal (AME) church that his family attended in Glen Cove. Camp Atwater was his first encounter with Black children playing the dozens, the game in which children can at once humorously, competitively, and cruelly give their opinions of each other and of each other's families. Camp Atwater also afforded Chet contact with older Black males. At the end of each Atwater summer, the good swimmers always took on the challenge to swim 3.5 miles. Chet and Clifton Wharton, who later became a well-known and distinguished African American leader, were the only two junior campers to receive a coveted award. Chet got his for being the only junior to complete the swim that summer. Such achievements stood him in good stead, as he had to contend with the tracks that had been left so indelibly by Samuel.

Young Samuel was nicknamed Ace, a sobriquet that had apparently been energetically earned and just as enthusiastically welcomed. Chet genuinely felt that Ace was a superior brother and human being. Chet knew that teachers "always read Ace's papers first so as to know how to set the curve." Ace was not only "superbly confident" but a very supportive brother. He set the tone for games played in the house, and his siblings looked to him for leadership and guidance. He was an obviously positive role model for Chet in many ways, such as leading Chet to conclude that he just *had* to do his homework. On the other hand, Chet also knew that he couldn't match the exploits of Ace, a childhood recognition that must, at least occasionally, have provoked some frus-

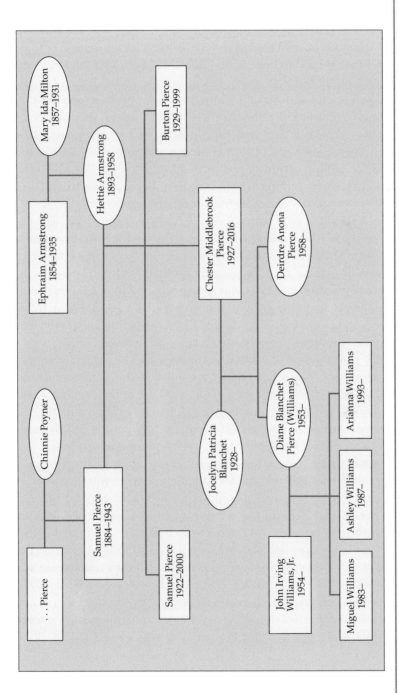

The family tree of Chester Middlebrook Pierce.

tration or anger. However, Chet could not recall a single fight with Ace during those growing-up years. On the contrary, Ace remained a reference point in music, sports, and academics, and he was the acknowledged leader because of his age as well as his achievements.

I still find it hard to believe that Ace and Chet never had even one significant tussle, but Chet insists this is the case. I think back, of course, to my own family and recall well my two older brothers mixing it up one Sunday morning. I remember clearly that my mother stopped it and delivered punishment with the old-fashioned stick she used when cooking Barbadian dishes that required a strong turning movement, such as the yellow cornmeal she turned into coo-coo. But Chet obviously started early learning how to avoid—or perhaps how to contain—the contentiousness that results from competitiveness.

Chet's strong urge to emulate Ace partially accounted for his hanging around with Ace's friends. But it was also no doubt made easier by Chet's big size. At one point, Chet was a full foot taller and about a hundred pounds heavier than his younger brother, Burton. The 2-year age gap between Burton and Chet was exacerbated by their unusual difference in size, so hanging out with Burton was not a good option. By the time he was 13 years old, Chet had reached his full height at well over 6 feet, which obviously provided him some advantages.

In the Caribbean of the 1940s, firstborn males in particular still enjoyed enormous prestige, no doubt a cultural tidbit passed on by the British. Some of those eldest sons made good use of their unique standing, much the way Chet's brother Ace did. In my family, the firstborn of six siblings seemed to understand instinctively what the British meant by duty and reason. He studied hard, won academic scholarships, took to foreign languages like a duck to water, made brilliant use on the playing field of his natural physical coordination, was a treble soloist in the island's cathedral choir, and still found time to be a Sea Scout of no mean distinction. I was thankful I was the third child. Comparison with the impressive achievements of a firstborn can make the youngsters wither. And in those days, unsophisticated West Indian parents had no clue that there was any clever skill to rearing children. All they understood was that the eldest child had charted a course to be followed relentlessly by all who came behind. In such a context, being a second-born was akin to at least a 10-year term of unwitting psychological harassment, of unceasing comparison with an elder brother who was almost always doing things right.

The age difference between Chet and his friends eventually led to his comeuppance. It happened one day when some of the boys started planning a beach party that included girls. However, the boys made it plain that youngsters—like Chester—were not welcome. Not that they told him he couldn't come; he just realized the rules didn't include extending him an invitation. His precocious growth spurt had allowed him to skip certain stages of childhood game-playing, so that, for example, he never learned to shoot marbles with any dexterity. But when at age 13 he was excluded from the beach party, he made a conscious decision to seek out his own age group. This lesson about being excluded ever so gently and its accompanying sensitivity to the rules of social etiquette are themes that would later emerge in Chet's professional thinking.

Chet entered Glen Cove High School's ninth grade at age 13 and graduated 4 years later, in 1944, leaving an impressive sports and academic record behind him. He lettered in football, basketball, and track, and as a senior, he played on the football team that won the New York State Championship. This performance earned him a place in Glen Cove City's Sports Hall of Fame, and old-timers talked of a special block that Chester had made in a particular football game. (Good old Ace had made the Hall of Fame several years before the city fathers decided that Chet's performance merited recognition.) Chet also recalled that throughout high school he was doing a lot of part-time work, so he had sufficient money to buy clothes and to go into New York City to see shows that held special interest for him. Moreover, he was the chief messenger for the whole city of Glen Cove in their civil defense system and had frequent drills with the head air-raid wardens.

Chet was always quite aware of Blacks' presence in Glen Cove. His mother maintained connections to her Southern roots, and there were numerous family friends who were transplants from the South. Many of these people were a part of the servant class in Glen Cove who were aspiring to better their lot. The Baptist and AME churches were the two Black religious centers in Glen Cove that sponsored picnics and other social events for the town's Black population, and Chet's mother played a prominent part in these goings-on. Indeed, Chet never went to a Sunday movie until well after he was married, believing all the time that to do so on the Lord's day would have been a serious contravention of God's preference.

His senior year in high school was full of events with a certain historic significance for Chet. His father died in November 1943, just before Thanksgiving and before Chet would play in an important championship football game. It was also the year Chet would be elected president of the senior class, the first Black in the history of Glen Cove to have that honor, and one particular honor that Ace had never won. It was the academic year when Chet would accept Harvard College's offer over those from Brown, Dartmouth, and the University of Pennsylvania—a decision that he thinks his father died too soon to have known.

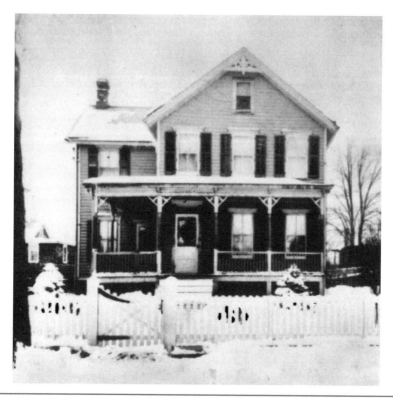

The Pierce family residence, Glen Cove, Long Island, circa 1940.

Chet worked hard at being senior class president, developing the yearbook, organizing parties for the class, and even raising money for the war effort. He recollects that because of his accomplishments as an underclassman teachers had named him to the nominations committee in charge of the elections for senior class president. Chet had suspicions about this maneuver, thinking it was a device to keep him from running. But a girl on the nominating committee proposed he run for the post, and he won the race without looking back. The teaching staff also appointed him to be stage manager for the senior play, a move he thought was meant to include him in the production, because a Black wouldn't compete for a dramatic role. These were minor, race-based, but still memorable encounters with which he was already learning to cope.

The female lead in the senior play was a White doctor's daughter who organized a party to be held at her house after the play. She offered Chet a special invitation, explaining to him that she had discussed the whole thing with her parents and they were in agreement with her notion that there would be no party if Chet declined to come. He acknowledges accepting the touching invitation and going to the party but doesn't recall anything about the party itself. Still, recognition of the gulf between the races in Glen Cove, where there was no formal racial segregation, was etched in his mind. He attended the senior prom with a Black male friend and two young Black women from New York City. After the prom, they went to a roadside restaurant for a meal, but they were refused service because the restaurant didn't serve Blacks. At the prom, he and a White female had agreed to dance together, a very daring thing even in Glen Cove of those days. Although nothing of any significance occurred as a result of the dance, it stays fixed in Chet's mind as a symbol of his resistance to the race-based differences that permeated Glen Cove.

These differences didn't go unnoticed in the Pierce household. For one thing, his father had always counseled his sons never to have their photographs taken with their arms around a White woman. He had also told them that it was a dangerous thing to be Black, and they ought never to be surprised by the treachery of Whites. Apparently, no one ever asked the senior Samuel what his experiences were that led him to such a cautious stance regarding Black-White relationships. It is also not clear whether it was what he saw daily at the White country club that had taught him so effectively or whether the past in Virginia still haunted him. But as an adolescent, Chester recognized the ambivalence evoked in himself by being around White girls. He had clandestine meetings with females from school, and when as a senior he had access to a car, it was even easier to go out with them. They liked Chet, no doubt because of his physical maturity as well as his distinguished accomplishments in school. Also, by then, his height had eliminated his obesity.

Chet tells the bittersweet story of a White schoolmate who told everybody she was in love with Mr. X. She had also secretly confided to Chet that he was the unidentified individual. As would be expected, the boys started working hard to figure out who Mr. X could possibly be. They quickly concluded that X simply could not be Chet, who in turn was struck by the White boys' arrogant assumption that their principal competitor could not be Black. But surprisingly, in those early years, Chet still did nothing to capitalize on this attraction between him and his White female schoolmates, even after he realized full well that some of them seemed "bold and brazen" and would seek him out to "accidentally" brush against him. Given this backdrop, it was an understandable game of fantasy that Chet and two Black buddies played one day when they just sat down and "divided" all the White girls in the school among them. They then assured each other that theoretically there were enough girls to go around, and there was no need for much struggle over the division. Curiously, the few Black girls in the school evoked little interest, although the reasons for this remain unclear and unstated. None of this diminished Chet's understanding that his father felt White women spelled trouble. There was also no doubt in Chet's mind that both of his parents would have conceived only of his marrying a black woman, even though Chet was surprised some years later to hear his mother supporting a cousin's decision to marry a White suitor. Interracial sexuality was certainly an American dilemma in the 1940s. Parental cautions in the midst of Chet's being around numerous White women must have caused substantial pressure in a virile adolescent trying to come to terms with his emerging sexuality, particularly because he was aware of the young White women's interest in him.

My early memories of contacts with White females provide substantial contrast. There were no Whites, male or female, in my local Barbadian neighborhood. And I attended all-male schools until I reached the university. Furthermore, my church choir was male, as was my scout troop. In colonial Barbados, therefore, I had no venue providing interaction with White girls. Neither my parents nor anyone else counseled me to be careful about social encounters with White women. In those days, it just wasn't done, although everybody knew that the Barbados plantation was a milieu for the quiet interplay of White men and Black women. In the logic of the day, however, that was miles away from a Black male youngster having anything to do with a White girl.

Although Chet's father worked 6 days a week, he still had a tremendous impact on the household. He was a family man who did his earnest best to make sure his children and wife never lacked for material things, even in the midst of the depression years. Samuel Pierce suffered from heart disease and possibly hypertension, and he had a strong feeling that he would die before reaching an advanced age. Chet remembers that his father went away twice to rest and recuperate when Chet was young, once to Bermuda and another time to Cuba.

Samuel did not work on Mondays. That was the day he went to Harlem to have his hair cut and to supervise his investments. On other evenings, he would sit without interruption in a little room at home and tidy up the accounts of his personal laundry business. It is an intriguing possibility that Samuel Pierce, born in 1884, might have had a parent who was born a slave. It is further noteworthy that there is no record of his having had any significant formal education, so what he achieved economically seems little short of miraculous. He owned the house his family occupied in a White neighborhood of Glen Cove and held property in other parts of the town. He also bought two apartment houses in upper Harlem and had the clever business insight to have them owned by corporations that he and his wife controlled. He took the further precaution of having the property managed by a White agent because he thought that widespread knowledge of his realty holdings might lead unnecessarily to legal hassles with both Whites and Blacks. Samuel Pierce also sought advice from a White lawyer and accountant to make sure that his investments were well protected. When he died in 1943, he left an elaborate will providing for both his wife and the education of his three children. He also had studied books on stocks and bonds and drew up written advice on companies in which his sons might usefully invest.

Today, Chet laughs at the fact that he didn't follow his father's business advice. But once the laughter's over, I recognize the potential importance of Chet's ignoring the emphasis that Samuel had placed on money. Chet's father had clearly understood that the fiscal imperative had to be a priority in the life of Black people. Samuel's own observations at the country club; the subsequent establishment of his shoeshine, cleaning, and laundry business; and his creative acquisition of property, stocks, and bonds point to a studied appreciation of how helpful it was for Black people to have money. In fact, Chet's own elaboration of his father's educational expectations for his children underscores Samuel's obvious linkage of money to the potential fulfillment of his dreams. So Samuel wasn't joking when he talked of stocks, bonds, and realty investments. But money lit no fire in Chet; it was no cardinal principle, no major base on which he would found his life structure. Other principles would later emerge that Chet would have no difficulty in attributing to his father. But as we shall see, Chet raised this idea of ignoring money to a veritable art form over the years when he consistently avoided ever seriously negotiating his salary; similarly, he accepted whatever he was offered to give a lecture. In a business sense, he never learned to set a price on his ideas or on his time.

I wonder what Chet's wife must have felt about his clear disdain of things fiscal. It is curious how often men of principle relegate money to a position of secondary importance. My father did it, with six children to feed, and my mother quietly told me from time to time how she could never understand my father's unwillingness to recognize what money could buy—things like food, clothes, education. My father always countered that God would provide those elements as a reward for the centering of one's life on Him. My mother answered that God never expected people on Earth to pass up opportunities He had placed there for them. For her, that was what life was all about, keeping one's eye on God and the chances He gave you to make good. I expect this argument gets played out in families all over the world—how to integrate economic self-sufficiency and other important life principles. And I have never found a way out of the dilemma created when men of principle insist that their families must live by values that clearly do not serve the families' interests.

Samuel Pierce also routinely gave counsel to his sons on other subjects. While taking a shave, he frequently called one of them and started one of his sessions of fatherly advice. He talked of how he thought American society would evolve and elements that were going to be important in determining anyone's success. He certainly made it clear that education was an absolute necessity, and in the Pierce household, the goal for the boys of going to college was simply not open to question. Samuel lectured his sons about the kind of woman they should marry, advising them to be careful in their choices. She didn't have to be rich, but she should be educated and able to care for the family. She didn't have to be pretty, but she should be nice enough to be introduced to a leading figure in her spouse's life. As a result of this wise counsel, Chet thinks all the Pierce boys "married up."

Samuel Pierce warned his sons they shouldn't get into any trouble with the law while they were accompanied by Whites because in those cases Blacks always received a significantly harsher punishment. He saw his sons as being the type who would attract women, a fact of life that required them to exercise good judgment in their dealings with the fairer sex. He wanted them to be always supportive of each other and of their mother, but without ceding their independence or allowing themselves to be taken advantage of.

Samuel Pierce was a "clothes horse" and obviously felt that being sartorially decked out helped make the man. He regularly took a bath in the late evening after his return from work, got dressed in his ascot and silk smoking jacket, and sat down to dine by himself. He was attuned to the fashion of the day and told his sons what clothes to wear and where to buy them. This was yet another arena where Chester concedes, with some obvious regret, he consistently ignored his father's advice. Samuel's sensitivity to the art of dressing probably helped him figure out the process he used to shine white shoes. He was successful enough in marketing this idea to have customers from all over the United States and even overseas send him their white shoes. The cleaning process involved Samuel's preparation and application of a special paste to the shoes. Then the shoes were delicately warmed in an oven. This was a domain where Samuel Pierce was very serious. He constantly used the metaphor of a certain person, whom we'll call here Giles Winston, as a reference point in talking about the symbolic interconnection between clothes and achievement, dress and class. Through constant contact, Samuel had taught many rich White men, such as Winston, how to dress and act. Since the Pierce boys had the same teacher, they could learn to dress and act the same way. Then, once they took education seriously, the elements would come together. They would be intellectually and externally prepared. Presumably, by extension, they would fit comfortably into any of the situations the White world would let them into. It seems at least inductively obvious that Samuel Pierce was preparing his sons for more than the society of Blacks. Indeed, while being clear about his identity as a Black man, he also warned them about a certain divisiveness that existed in the Black community and about the possibility of treachery from Blacks.

Samuel Pierce's cautious nature extended to a variety of subjects. He thought a husband ought never to tell his wife how much money he had; husbands, not wives, should control the household funds. He believed that it was generally impossible for a man and his wife to love each other equally. Consequently, it would generally lead to a better outcome if the woman's love were stronger. A man who loved more ended up often being "henpecked." With this brand of early-twentieth-century machismo being exhibited by his father, Chet still doubts that the senior Samuel had time to engage in any extramarital affairs because he worked so many hours. Chet also makes the point that his mother shared his father's life strategy, especially because Samuel was clearly family oriented and also so very supportive of his wife's role not only within the family but also in the broader society.

Samuel was enthusiastic about using role models as a way of teaching his children what the world offered and what it was possible for Blacks to achieve. During his Monday excursions into Harlem, he often met college athletes who were waiting to have their hair cut. Samuel would invite these struggling but competitive young men to his home for dinner so that his own sons could have the chance to rub shoulders with a class of persons who were displaying initiative and potential for success. In the same spirit, Samuel took Chet from time to time to the country club where he worked. Chet recalls seeing Fats Waller entertain at the club and specifically has the memory of that famous musician entering the club through its front door. That was a significant act in those days because as a matter of custom Blacks did not use the club's front entrance. Samuel, of course, seized the opportunity to point out to Chet that Whites will give Blacks a lot of latitude if the Black individual in question has exploitable skills and can do something well.

The country club played an important role in Samuel's life, and it is where he found the idea for Chet's first and middle names. Henry Middlebrook Crane was a member of the club and the Massachusetts Institute of Technology benefactor who designed the Pontiac automobile. The name Chester came from a Black lawyer, Chester Crumpler, who worked at the club to earn money for his education after having served as an officer in World War I.

It is hard for me to let go this image of the club, the country club, the place where others hang out and you can't go. I had more than a passing acquaintance with the club metaphor, growing up in British-dominated Barbados in the forties and fifties. For me, it was particularly the Aquatic Club, where Whites alone went and Black Barbadians stood on the outside, quietly contemplating what it really meant that they didn't—or couldn't—belong to this apparently select institution. When one is on the outside looking in, with one's view at least partially obscured or skewed, it is hard to avoid inventing one's own private images of what goes on inside the club. But Samuel Pierce was in a different position. Although he obviously did not belong to the club and could not claim membership in it, he knew what went on inside. This was very special knowledge, and he put it to good use.

I have long been persuaded that the club was one of the most pervasive and influential metaphors in Barbadian colonial society. Clubs and the club mentality were at the core of British colonial psychology. Besides the Aquatic Club, Whites also had the Royal Yacht Club for sailing and the Savannah Club for tennis. They even managed to have separate church services, through the custom of attending the matins service in the island's churches, leaving evening for the rest of the population. It was a way of guarding their special space. It is natural to think that the purpose of those clubs was to keep out the Barbadians. But I think the Whites also wanted to keep themselves in, proximately linked, their cultural views unadulterated by the intoxicating and seductive ways of black Barbados. Even today, the White and monied groups in Barbados are still preoccupied with the club metaphor. Several of the island's most select hotels, for instance, still have mechanical barriers that force all automobiles to stop, thereby requiring an interaction between driver and the hotel's security guard. Some say the mechanical barriers are there to enhance security. I say the barrier is meant to promote difference, to foster the club ambience, to make every black Barbadian think twice about whether Barbadians belong in the precincts of White affluence.

It seems likely that Samuel was himself intrigued by the affiliative possibilities of the club. He was a member of the Masonic Order, and he told his sons about the organizations they should join, recommending particularly that they should become members of fraternities once they were in college. As a result, Chet and his two brothers all joined the Black fraternity Alpha Phi Alpha in their collegiate years. Their father thought fraternity membership would provide a necessary social credential and would facilitate their establishing networks. Chet later joined Nu Sigma Nu, the oldest (and at the time, all-White) medical school fraternity, but not without some minor trauma once again. The national office threatened to expel the Harvard chapter when it announced that the chapter intended pledging Chet and another Black student. The chapter went ahead anyway, and the national office backed down.

Curiously enough, Chet never became a Mason like his father, partly because his father apparently never recommended membership in the Masonic Order. However, Samuel understood well the significance of networking and saw it as a feasible and useful task, even for someone occupying his position in an all-White context. It is clear he purposefully cultivated certain relationships, and this permitted him later on to boast to Chet that through judicious use of his contacts it would take him only about 24 hours to reach the President of the United States. This had to have been one direct benefit of having physical access to the inside of the club, even without the status of membership.

Chester Pierce has multiple and different images of his father: teaching Chester how to box; playing golf and tennis; hugging Chester and reading to him as a youngster, from a kind of children's book called a Big Little Book; visiting Chester's school to check on how he was doing; generously giving money to Chet, even though Samuel would then mark every cent he spent in a book he kept for that purpose; never muzzling his wife in any exchange or dispute. Chet has no memory of paternal cruelty; even at my insistence, he cannot recall his father's angry moments. And in defense against my obvious disbelief, Chet explains that his own wife has pointed out to him that he has almost certainly borrowed from his father the technique of avoiding anger and withdrawing at moments when it is imperative to confront the serious and the difficult. In a further attempt to consolidate this theme of the nurturing and comforting father, Chet underlines the idea that corporal correction fell to his mother, and he is unable to evoke even a flickering association of his father and any sense of personal humiliation. It is almost too good to be true. This notion of a strong, thoughtful, caring, and ever-present Black father is one that has evoked considerable lay and professional analysis in the last two decades. Certainly, it is a characteristic that immediately sets Chester Pierce's family apart from many present-day Black families. But additionally, for Samuel never to have been the source of Chet's hurt or anger is, at the least, I think, unusual.

My own father was also strong, thoughtful, caring, and very much present in the life of the family. But I know of no Barbadians of my generation who avoided at least one morning when cane or belt met backside and a child rushed off to school or church in a torrent of confusion and tears, demeaned and hurting and aghast that loving parents could be so amazingly unfair. In fact, in my day, youngsters worked hard to avoid encountering the principle of double jeopardy: some Barbadian parents were not above flogging their child and then later asking the schoolmaster to add some additional corporal punishment so that the child could clearly understand the gravity of his or her transgressions. Samuel had to have been much before his time, so full of insight.

But there may be another explanation for Samuel's unwillingness to hurt his sons. And I wonder about Samuel's own experiences of profound pain—which must have existed, but about which we know so little. Chester Pierce knows, too, that there are some unexplained gaps here. For example, his father never talked about any demeaning experiences occurring at the club where he worked. He also never discussed his own relatives. At home, there was a picture of Chet's paternal grandmother but none of his paternal grandfather; Chet never knew either of them. He still can't be rid of the nagging idea that his father had an unhappy and deprived childhood, which would partly explain Samuel's profound reticence regarding his early years. But I also theorize that Samuel thought it useful to keep his pain private, to protect his children from trauma and to be as rarely as possible the source of any of their suffering.

Musing about fathers often raises issues of comparison and competition, and Chet also feels that urge. He concludes that his father was, indeed, a special man, and he pauses over the worrisome thought that he hasn't done much with the "superb jump start" his father gave him. In the economic arena, the comparison is most readily palpable; Chet is sure he didn't accomplish fiscally as much as he should have. But he talks in a contemplative fashion about not having made a more "dramatic contribution" to medicine or to some other area of activity, of missing the chance to leave a greater and more lasting legacy. He characterizes his contributions to psychiatry as not being "timeless" and points out he has done nothing that will last forever. In referring to the many honors he has received, including the 1995 induction as an Honorary Fellow into Britain's Royal College of Psychiatrists, Chet thinks that once one lives long enough a certain number of deserved and undeserved honors will come. Still, he is thankful that he didn't waste all the opportunities provided by the efforts of his father and concedes that he was also limited by his own personality and character. "Life might have been different had I been more aggressive here, worked harder there, or spent more time on this or that."

But with obvious pride, he recalls the elegance of his father's lifestyle and his joy of living. Chet thinks it is one of the tricks of fate that Samuel Pierce could not have been the famous "Mr. Winston." Had he been, "he would have done it right. If he'd been lord of the manor, he'd have done it right. He had style and panache." Chet also credits his father with having inculcated in him articles of faith and a sense of hope, in spite of all the misfortune and treachery in the surrounding society. I cannot resist reflecting on my own father, particularly because the wound caused by his death is still raw, and I feel so much sympathy and respect for Chet's attempts to come to terms with his father's life and legacy.

My own father was a slim, handsome, articulate Barbadian who found pleasure in his island roots and knew full well the impact of his personal charm on those around him. Stories have it that he gave his own father hell while growing up; but he settled down in his early adulthood, once he found the church and married my mother. He was also a local politician at the parish level and probably would have made a name in national island politics if he hadn't aligned himself with the wrong political party. This was a sin in small Caribbean islands, and his peers never forgave him. So he eventually immigrated to the United States in 1956 with his family and turned to his work as a preacher. When he retired and returned to Barbados in the 1980s, he reveled in his status as a returned son who was by then independent of local power politics. And he enjoyed his prestige as a senior pastor who was considered brilliant in the pulpit.

Chet's mother, Hettie Armstrong Pierce, was her own woman, and she left her distinctive and indelible mark on Chet. We know she was born in 1893 and grew up in North Carolina. After her 1909 marriage to Samuel Pierce, she moved to Glen Cove, Long Island. It is much easier for Chet to trace her roots, as we have seen. Chet can provide no information about the sociocultural context that allowed Hettie's phenotypically White father, with blond hair and blue eyes, to court Hettie's more Native American–looking mother. But Hettie identified her own persona as Black and lived out this identification most clearly, while at the same time letting it be known she was not the descendant of slaves.

Hettie was energetic and took an intense interest in local organizations. She was politically active and pugnaciously awaited the opportunity when someone would offend her so that she could move swiftly to correct the offender. Chet recalls her as feisty and readily militant, qualities that underscore her sense of justice and a willingness to stand up for her rights. Hettie took Chet along when she once visited the tearoom at a department store, either Gimbels or Macy's, just to see whether they would serve her. Chet cannot recall the outcome of the visit, although he can see vividly Hettie's determination to test the system. Chet relates how, after her husband died, Hettie went to work as a housekeeper for the famous photographer Francesco Scavullo. This man found out that he had more than a simple housekeeper in Hettie. She was influential and imposing; she knew what she wanted and how she wished it done.

Scavullo confirmed that Hettie worked for him between 1948 and 1954. They met when Hettie and one of her friends visited his photography studio. The friend had been recommended to Scavullo as a potential employee, but it turned out that she had no time for the job. On the other hand, Hettie, who by that time had already mourned her husband and sent her three sons off to college, was available. A remarkable relationship then developed. Scavullo recalled her as a woman who dressed simply and who was impeccably clean and neat. She was motherly, protective, very strong, and well organized. When she worked for him, she stayed in New York City with a friend and returned to Glen Cove on weekends.

Chet loved to eat his mother's cooking, which no doubt contributed to his early childhood obesity. Besides her culinary excellence, Chet also remembers her green thumb, which was well reflected in the impressive gardens that adorned both the front and rear yards, and through which she let her neighbors know of her intention to be competitive. Hettie could sew and do needlepoint, and she loved parlor games. She also raised money for her church and had a strong commitment to helping others. She was a radio fan, keeping abreast of her radio serials and rooting vigorously for the Brooklyn Dodgers during baseball season.

Chet sees Hettie in his mind's eye as being generous, and he describes his mother's Halloween practice of buying napkins and baking pastry, then tying together little gift bags and distributing them, along with money and candy, to children in the neighborhood. Then, at Christmas, Hettie baked many fruitcakes for friends and others she thought would appreciate them. In general, Hettie was also the disciplinarian in the family, keeping the household straight and orderly. Chet views her as the keeper of moral values and the teacher of routine household manners and etiquette. It was she who made it clear that Chet could entertain girls at home, but only when Hettie was there to provide the appropriate supervision. She mixed her strictness with lots of hugging and petting of Chet, indulging many of his wants and calling him "Baby Boy." She was constant in her emphasis on ethics and politeness and her attention to social values. It was Hettie who insisted that thank-you notes be written to anyone who had been kind to her sons.

Hettie's personal confidence was reflected in the proud way she carried herself. She talked a lot about race matters and Black heroes such as Paul Robeson and Marcus Garvey, as well as the role of Black soldiers in America's wars. She complained that Negroes in the North weren't agitating enough, and she was irritated by the notion that progress for Blacks had come through leadership from Southerners or from West Indians. She wanted all Blacks to be contributors to Black progress, to have special regard for education, and to stand up to Whites. However, it was Samuel who maintained the family's collection of books on Black history, such as the work of Carter G. Woodson.

It is curious to me that my own mother was in some ways much more sedate and conservative than my father, while in other ways she was the more practical of the two. She had more fiscal savvy but was never interested in confronting the colonial practices that had kept down so many Barbadians of her generation. Still, she believed earnestly, and agreed with my father, that education was a cardinal factor in the future of her children.

With their different personality styles, Hettie and Samuel Pierce came together in their collective emphasis on certain issues that they saw as the bedrock of their family. They constantly focused on the interaction between Blacks and Whites, with hardly a day passing without some discussion of White people. Chet heard how dangerous it was to be Black, and his parents inculcated in him very early the basic idea that White decision-makers rarely considered Blacks before reaching important policy conclusions. Moreover, Hettie and Samuel were persuaded that highly visible Blacks always ran the risk of eventual persecution and that Blacks needed to be constantly aware of the fragility of Black-White relationships.

At this point, Chet becomes pensive and remarks almost apologetically that were Hettie and Samuel still alive today, they would see Ace's public legal difficulties as proof once again that one ought never to be surprised by Whites' betrayal of Blacks. (Ace was under investigation for allegedly using his influence illegally to help others while he was Secretary of Housing and Urban Development under President Reagan.) Such experiences, coupled with the repetitive teachings of his parents, still make it difficult for Chet to ascertain, in his interactions with any given White person, whether that person is behaving as an individual or as a representative of the White collective. Hettie and Samuel understood this distinction because they had to put trust in White lawyers and accountants in order to protect their personal finances.

Hettie clearly was a homemaker and the disciplinarian who raised the children while Samuel worked long hours to support his family and a lifestyle that included the wearing of distinctive smoking jackets. Chet thinks that his father was most likely a conservative Republican, but

Hettie was an activist and a Democratic loyalist who helped to organize the NAACP in Glen Cove. They had both come to some agreement on how they wanted their children to grow up, and they jointly predicted the racial obstacles they felt their children would face. Both parents were fierce in teaching that their children were as good as everyone else, often using the metaphor of Giles Winston, whom Samuel in reality encountered regularly at his club. The parents also provided Black newspapers in the home, such as the *Norfolk Journal and Guide*, *Baltimore Afro-American*, *Pittsburgh Courier*, and *New York Amsterdam News*, in addition to many other magazines and books. Some of the literature came from the club where Samuel worked, but most was bought.

In many respects, of course, the Pierce family was quite fortunate, and in looking back, Chet can think of only a few incidents that caused substantive stress in the years before he left home and went off to university. When he was about 4 years old, he was playing in a child's wagon on a downhill slope and lost control of it. In the ensuing accident, he lost consciousness for about 12 hours before waking up in a hospital. Although he never experienced any more problems from the accident, it obviously caused his family considerable fright.

The other significant event in Chet's memory was his father's death, which took place close to Thanksgiving Day in 1943. The senior Samuel was hospitalized about 10 days before ultimately dying of congestive heart failure. Chet's football team dedicated one of their last games to the honor of Samuel Pierce. Chet feels confident that racism played no part in influencing the medical care his father received while he was hospitalized. Samuel anticipated his death and told the family that life should go on. So Chet continued to go to school and to work part-time at his father's country club in the locker room and shining shoes. Ace returned to his post in the military, and their mother did her best to care for Burton and to keep her own life structured and orderly.

Chet thinks Hettie did change somewhat after his father's passing. For one thing, within a few months she developed diabetes mellitus. But a more profound change could be seen in her bearing, as if she had lost a certain confidence and sprightliness. Chet recalls Hettie's instructing him to carry out some task during this period; instead of doing it snappily, he objected and told Hettie that his father would never have insisted that he do what she was asking. Rather than standing her ground, Hettie just gave in, something that would simply have been unthinkable in the period before Samuel's death. Hettie never remarried, and Chet couldn't recall her having any serious suitors, although he thought there may have been a few men around expressing an interest in her for the material things she had. Hettie did have two sisters and nephews and nieces living in the Glen Cove area who undoubtedly provided her moral support.

Chet took to heart his father's recommendation to get on with his life. He didn't cry at the funeral because "men don't cry," but he thought about his father for years. Long after Samuel's passing, Chet would complain around Thanksgiving time about not feeling very good. This "anniversary response" was characterized by a sensation of indifference, slowing down, lassitude, and decreased energy that would last until Christmas before tapering off and ultimately disappearing.

At the time of his father's death, Chet was in his final year of high school and therefore contemplating going to college. This had been a step often discussed in his household, and Chet saw applying to college as an exercise akin to seeking a driver's license. By that time, of course, Ace had long since gone off to Cornell. His parents had always talked of college, and Chet's mother discouraged his dream of going to Stanford because she thought it was too far away. Plans were being made for him to go to Dartmouth when his Latin teacher suggested he apply to Harvard. He did it all mechanically, without understanding much about difficulties inherent in the application process or its competitive features. In assessing his readiness for admission, he thinks his qualifications were obvious: an A average, presidency of the senior class and election to numerous other positions, participation in varsity athletics, competency with different musical instruments and membership in several music groups, community service activities, and involvement in work on weekends and in the summers. So the acceptance letters came, and he chose Harvard only because the school principal previously had suggested, sympathetically, that he might not be accepted to Harvard.

Ace had played a role in the application process and had approved all the college choices. Cornell was, quite naturally, eliminated because Chet couldn't stand the thought of competing with Ace's record in athletics and scholarship on the famed Ithaca campus. So Chet prepared for Harvard, without even giving a thought to how the university fees would be paid. He just knew it was not a problem because his father had long ago provided for this next step in Chet's development. Hettie was not a major part of this psychological preparation either because she was busy completing business related to her husband's death. In addition, she was preoccupied by Ace. By that time, Ace was working in army criminal investigations, and his whereabouts were hard to track. No doubt, having just lost her husband, and with the European war on everybody's mind, she was imagining dire things happening to Ace. Still, Hettie found the time to knit things for Chet to take to college.

In retrospect, Chet finds this transition fairly unremarkable and very much a matter of course. He relates it partly to his ignorance of the complexity and the inherent difficulties of the passage from high school to university. Besides, everybody had prepared for his eventual going away to college. He recalls no inkling of his mother's being sad at his leaving, and saying good-bye to Burton occupies no prominent place in his memory. The parting from family at this juncture was inevitable. Its natural and apparently easy, sequential occurrence forces Chet into further contemplation of his status as a young Black man in 1944 off to one of the premier educational institutions in the country. It brings to his mind the concept of a *supernormal childhood*, an idea with which he is familiar in his work with astronauts and that describes an individual who has done the right thing at the right time in perfect sequence.

I remain aggressively curious about the elements that may have facilitated such supernormal development in Chet's case. He responds with a list worth noting: his family was not poor; he had no juvenile gangs to contend with; he was in contact with other boys who in their own heads entertained no thoughts destined to get them into trouble; he enjoyed a stable home with dependable brothers; he had the constant and loving presence of two parents who were accepting and supportive and who anticipated his wants; he lived in a neighborhood that was forward-looking and generally not hostile toward him; it was a given in his home that acquiring a university education was an important objective; there were constant and powerful messages from a father who insisted that his children, like Giles Winston, could go anywhere in the world; and his family recognized that economic security was an important ticket to success in any society, Black or White.

I marvel at Chet's level of emotional containment, both then and now, his luck in receiving the cards life dealt him so early in the game. His mother didn't try to keep her special baby boy at home to compensate for the profound loss she suffered with Samuel's death. And Chet had managed to escape all the tempting emotional entanglements that often work to keep adolescents away from the task of pursuing their studies at a distant educational institution.

Thinking about Chet's preoccupation with race matters during his adult career prompted me on repeated occasions to verify that I had missed no particular event in his adolescent or childhood years that symbolized bold, blatant, raw racial discrimination—something that would make current-day commentators raised on the diet and vocabulary of posttraumatic stress disorder jump to their feet screaming that the experience of racial injustice is what rendered Chet so hypersensitive to the matter of race. Then they might have chortled that such feelings are generally exacerbated by repeated interactions with a down-on-his-luck, angry, poorly performing Black father who blames his situation on "Mr. Charlie."

It turns out I missed no special event in Chet's early years. The elder Samuel Pierce did not deliver his lessons during bouts of despair. Instead, it seems he set about to establish himself as a nurturing and comforting provider-father so that he could teach Chet steadily that, in the real world, it *did* make a difference whether one was Black or White. Samuel made it clear to his sons that he had no faith in the law's intent to protect equally the interests of Blacks and Whites. He also encouraged his sons, with Hettie's support, to make men of themselves and to think of their future with undisguised hope. That is why he started them so early on the road to building connections to other achieving Blacks and, moreover, to thinking about establishing links to those Whites with power. Given Samuel's position at the country club, it had to be easy for him to imagine the possibility that the day might come for him or his sons when using such contacts would be necessary.

It is worth repeating how Chet recalled readily that in the Glen Cove period rarely a day passed without his parents talking about White folks. Their emphasis was on the notion that Blacks should never be surprised by the treachery of Whites. Paradoxically, his father, who worked in an all-White environment, never spoke at home of any experiences that could have been construed as demeaning or discriminatory. This led Chet to point out to me that his father liked to emphasize the potential strengths of his sons, not their weaknesses. Consequently, the paternal and maternal—but especially the paternal—warnings about White people were framed in a context of wily competition rather than in the more transparent fabric of red-hot racial hatred. Samuel and Hettie seemed to know they were preparing their children for a lifetime of unremitting struggle with Whites, not just for some ephemeral civil rights skirmish. These were, of course, the quite necessary fundamental lessons for a 17-year-old African American male to take with him as he left home for the very first time.

Two additional points are important here. First, Chet only obliquely frames the notion that his family represented the opposite of what sociologists now call the phenomenon of Black family disorganization or dislocation. But it is all the more remarkable, as one considers the origin and educational achievement of both Samuel and Hettie, that they both accomplished distinctive differentiation of their roles within the family; that they achieved a shared vision of what they wanted for their sons; and that they wanted to live out their dreams in a social context that was also highly organized. In other words, the neighborhood in which they deliberately chose to rear their children was experiencing relatively little social disorganization.

The second point is related to a philosophical stance that Chet has taken from time to time over the years, one whose basis I had never really grasped. Chet has a habit of saying, without much more, that Blacks ought to be constantly studying Whites. He generally intends us to understand the comment in the context where Blacks and Whites are often engaged in an interaction but with differing intended objectives. Listeners often hear the advice as a means of waging war competently. But I now understand it as a deformation of the more profound message formulated by Chet as a result of Samuel's teaching. And to deform the thesis is to miss the pervasive metaphor of the country club. Samuel recognized that having the opportunity to observe Whites was the best way to understand them, to be able ultimately to contend with them, to acquire the capacity to compete with them, and to anticipate their every move. This was not the simple gesture of waging war against Whites; it was the far more complicated task of pursuing peace with them, but on a basis that guaranteed or at least moved toward mutual respect and socioeconomic equity.

2

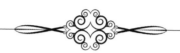

The Harvard Student Years

In 1944, World War II was still on and universities were open all year round. Chester Pierce didn't have to wait for fall; he took off for Harvard in the summer, going by train from New York City to Boston by himself. His mother had offered to accompany him, but he declined, fully aware that the whole family had driven Ace to Cornell some years earlier. Chet was moving on, and he was doing so alone and in his own way. On the train, he saw two young men he thought might also be going to Harvard. They acknowledged cordially, but stiffly, that they were in fact headed for Cambridge.

No longer in Glen Cove, Chet was just beginning to learn about the philosophy of difference. For instance, while waiting in the registration queue in Cambridge, he met several other young men and they all decided to hum some four-part Handel. They assigned parts to each other, and Chet faked his way through the tenor part. When he suddenly realized these chaps were serious, he found himself musing that Harvard was definitely not the kind of place he was accustomed to. It must have been quite a shock to suddenly encounter such talent among his peers. It certainly was unnerving to me in 1959 when I realized that a member of my Harvard freshman class was already a published author. In my case, I left Brooklyn for Harvard with a bit more ritual than Chet's venture. My father drove me up to Cambridge in his Chevrolet Biscayne with its Bahama-blue fins. We spent at least one night with some old Barbadian friends of his, a family who would provide solid community support throughout my Harvard stay. I took the trip regularly from Cambridge to the West Indian section of Boston on Sundays to eat Bajan dishes that would remind me of home and the fact that I was loved and had three Christian names full of purpose and tradition. But I had also left for Harvard fully dependent on scholarship help, without which I would have been unable to attend the university.

When Chet reported to Harvard's Lowell House, he was given a single room, something he realized later was quite unusual. But Master Perkins apparently had done it deliberately to avoid any problems and also to treat Chet with unmistakable deference. After a semester, two seniors invited him to move in with them, and he accepted. After those two graduated, other roommates joined him, and he remained in the same suite of rooms. His roommates over the years were a diverse group of people with different interests, backgrounds, and religions. He never lived with a Black student in those college years, although he recalled that at least one other Black man had lived in Lowell House and that there were a few Blacks in other residences on campus.

I had spoken to Chet earlier about my Lowell House years and thought it likely that I was less enthusiastic about my experiences there. However, I had actually enjoyed tremendously the interactions with other students, some of whom have remained very good friends over the past 60 years. But I now understand better my irritability with certain Lowell House faculty who evidently saw Harvard as their own private club and who did their best to make it clear that some students simply did not belong there. Still, my mother's advice often rang in my ears, and I kept in front of me the reason I was there. She had warned me not to be distracted by the silly preoccupations of provincial faculty. I was there for an education at a great university. Once I really internalized that idea, I enjoyed the place more and made excellent use of the experience.

During his first summer at Harvard, Chet practiced football with the team and played his first game in September. In that initial season, he was selected for the first team. Not surprisingly, being a varsity team member gave him considerable standing among his peers and made it easier for him to meet people. However, his popularity was occasionally marred by negative commentary. For instance, upon his entrance into the football stadium for the first game, he heard someone say, "There's a nigger." But on the whole, this experience was particularly uncharacteristic of his Harvard undergraduate days, which still evoke pleasant memories. He had lots of friends, and even people on the street would stop him to chat. With such good social support, he found it easy to maintain good grades throughout the 4 years.

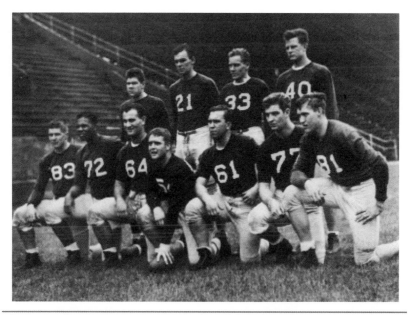

Chester Pierce (jersey 72), Harvard football team, 1944.

With all the new connections he had established at Harvard, Chet ventured home only for holidays; his mother visited him occasionally in Cambridge. The result was that they saw little of each other except in the summer. Mothers have always had this hardship to contend with, being separated from their children as they grow into adulthood. In Hettie's case, she had permanently lost the elder Samuel, her husband, and now her two older sons were out making their place in the world. At age 52, she was having to cope with these important losses while at the same time she had to concentrate on raising Burton, who was then about 16.

Meanwhile, Chet continued to make his way through Harvard with a certain distinctiveness. He played varsity football and lacrosse, and for part of one year he even added basketball to the list. His clearest memory of hardship in his undergraduate career was having to contend with spring football, lacrosse, organic chemistry, and comparative anatomy in the same semester. By the time he reached his final college year, he was elected to one of the three senior Marshal positions, the first time a Black man had been so honored in the history of Harvard. Later, this honor was amplified when the Class of 1948 had its twenty-fifth reunion, in 1973. The class donated a record total of about $1.1 million to the Harvard College Fund, earmarking part of the gift for scholarships to honor six people, among whom were Senator Robert Kennedy and Professors John Finley, Elliott Perkins, and Chester Pierce.

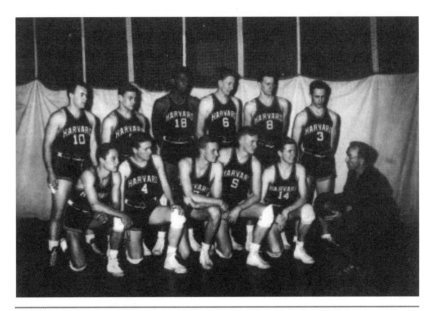

Chester Pierce (jersey 18), Harvard basketball team, 1945.

In the midst of such social, athletic, and educational success, Chet collected a number of negative race-related experiences that doubtless contributed to the development and evolution of his later views that racism was a primary construct that defined the etiquette of interaction among individuals in the United States. For example, at about two o'clock one morning, a White college classmate telephoned to tell him that a certain bar in Cambridge did not serve Blacks. The caller was outraged and insisted that something had to be done, so he and Chet agreed to prepare a story for the *Harvard Crimson*, the campus newspaper. Chet and his friends later came up with a plan. They decided that one of Chet's roommates would go first to the bar and seek admission. Of course, he was served. But when Chet entered and tried to be served, he was rejected. Then a second roommate entered, and he also was served.

After the story about the establishment's racist policies ran in the *Crimson*, with corroborating photos, students organized picket lines in front of the bar. Chet later heard that the bar owner had claimed untruthfully that Chet, who never smoked or drank, had been intoxicated and somewhat unruly, and that was why he had to be excluded from the bar. Chet also recounted an addendum to this story. Recently, he and his family went to visit Ed Davis, a White college roommate who had taken part in the newspaper plan. Ed reminded Chet that when the picket line was set up in front of the bar, a car drove by and a passenger shouted,

"You fucking nigger lovers, go to hell!" At the time of the incident, Chet told his roommate that he recognized the passenger as a Harvard student with whom he regularly ate lunch in a science laboratory. Chet was struck by the fact that he had blocked out this incident—and he continues to muse about the role of repression in coping with trauma related to racism. We both recognize the value of this selective, involuntary forgetting; the alternative is to chew on the insult until its harsh reality makes one's gums bleed. This rarely attenuates the pain. Furthermore, there is still the indignity of spitting out saliva that is tainted red, suggesting even to kind bystanders that you might be suffering from some malignant illness, being eaten away from the inside out and not fit to be around. That's what it does to you, ruminating about a racist insult. You end up being the punished victim. So why not forget the insult if you can, especially if it's small enough to swallow without causing your insides to act up and to make the unambiguous statement that they, too, have had enough.

In 1947, in his senior year, Chet traveled with the football team to play against the University of Virginia. Harvard had told Virginia in 1946 that it intended to have Chet Pierce make the trip. The Southern institution made it clear that Chet couldn't stay in the same hotel with his teammates; but in a conciliatory gesture, the university still provided a mansion where Chet could sleep. The Harvard coach sent the first two teams to stay in the mansion with Chet. But meals presented another problem because they were served only at the hotel and Chet was not allowed to go through the hotel's front door. Once again, the coach and the team stood by him, and they all went through the kitchen with their beleaguered teammate. When they finally took the field at game time, the coach was at Chet's side, setting himself up as a target for any missile intended for his Black player. Although Harvard lost that game badly, Chet has remained ever proud that Harvard stood its ground that time, when he was the first Black to play football in the South against a White team. The pattern was the same when he played lacrosse against the University of Maryland and Navy teams in Maryland. The Harvard team would buy takeout food so they could eat in the car with Chet, who still couldn't expect to be served in a Southern restaurant in the late 1940s.

The game against Virginia was apparently Harvard's first football trip to the South, and the event has been dutifully recorded in Harvard's annals, with the accompanying notation that Virginia won 47-0. However, Chet thinks it was mere capricious chance that he was a participant in that historic moment and sees no other particular contribution as deriving from him at that point. In his terms, he was practically a bystander, simply watching as history was being made.

I listen attentively to this kind of story because I never had that type of experience growing up—this reality of being told bluntly that I was not allowed to enter some place because I was Black. The British had a different way of doing things. For instance, I knew I was not welcome at the Aquatic Club. But in true English fashion, I wasn't excluded from the Club because of some legal rule. I knew it just wasn't done. It simply would have been unthinkable for me to have tried to get in there. This British colonial technique of establishing difference based on race is not the same as prosecuting difference with a racist vengeance. I think the two political approaches result in differing psychological impact, with blunt racism being by far the more malignant. Chet and I will doubtless return to this theme. But for the time being, I will not leave it with the hanging implication that West Indian Blacks are superior to American Blacks. Such intragroup competition may serve other interests but certainly not mine. Nevertheless, I think it significant that the experience of the overt and legally supported racist act is psychologically different from experiencing racial differentiation predicated on cultural rules. So I did not go to the Aquatic Club. But I had no trouble enrolling at the finest grammar school on the island because the entrance examination was based on merit. And no one ever told me or any other Black student that intellectual performance was linked to race. Of course, it is also true that Chet did not confront any such barriers in Glen Cove. Indeed, in those formative years, growing up in Glen Cove was closer to being reared in Barbados than it was to being raised in Maryland.

I must confess I am not confident that my view is universally held, even by my Black colleagues and friends. Frantz Fanon would most likely argue that the impact of the colonizer can certainly be, in some cases, quite malignant. I would not object firmly to that assertion. But I still think it is of substantial importance that I was not prevented from obtaining a first-class basic education in colonial Barbados.

When one of Chet's closest college friends from a very prominent family decided to get married in the South, the subject of his being invited to the wedding simply never arose. He claims he wasn't angry or bitter, because he knew the rules. But that's hard for me to accept so quickly, unless one grants that he means externally visible or obvious anger and bitterness. These minitraumas had to be powerful reminders that he was in some ways not quite a Harvard man in the fullest sense.

The paradoxical business of being found acceptable while still not being totally accepted haunted Chet in other areas as well. He had roommates who were members of private clubs at Harvard and who talked in front of him about keeping Jews out of their clubs. Still, the question of Chet's becoming a member of any club just never came up, and the general question of Blacks joining such clubs was not a topic of discussion. He concedes that in retrospect he regretted never having been invited to join the Hasty Pudding. That was a membership he thought he rightfully deserved because in those college days he was an excellent writer of music; had a solid interest in musical composition; and played a respectable piano, accordion, and trumpet. However, membership in the Hasty Pudding eluded him, as did a sense of total membership in the Harvard community.

In our continuing discussion of Blacks and the phenomenon of their belonging to predominantly White institutions, Chet always answers in terms of individuals and not in terms of institutions or organizations. This perspective permits him to show continued respect for groups and institutions like the Hasty Pudding and Harvard, while at the same time maintaining more pronounced suspicion of those individuals in the organizations who wreak microtrauma on minority people and sustain homogeneity of the institution. That is, of course, why Chet insists that over the years only a handful of Whites he has met have not generated suspicion.

It is possible that besides the urging from his father that he join a Black fraternity, the lack of an invitation to join any of the select White Harvard clubs made it easier for him to pledge the all-Black Alpha Phi Alpha. In the late 1940s, there was only a graduate chapter of the Alphas in Boston, and it was tottering. Luckily, several of their members had just returned from military service, and they decided to breathe life back into the chapter. Some of them recognized that admitting undergraduates directly into the Boston chapter would help renew its lease on life; and Chet was a beneficiary of this new policy. The group provided opportunities for a lively social life, and Chet latched onto the social structure provided by the Alphas.

I am reminded of my own refusal to join any Black fraternity when I was at Harvard in the early sixties because I found the violence and cruelty that were part of the hazing process to be unacceptable. I never could understand why I would have to undergo punishment so as to be persuaded of the reality of our Black brotherhood. When I ask Chet about this, he points out that he refused ever to be a part of the paddling, and he never participated in what he agrees were demeaning practices. I wish I could let go of it more easily. But I realize the depth of my offense at witnessing Blacks assault the minds and bodies of other Blacks. Black friends told me then, and some still tell me now, that the violence builds mental and physical toughness. I have never been persuaded. Nevertheless, I realize that I have always harbored strong feelings about Harvard's private clubs that systematically excluded Blacks.

And it rankled me as much that the Black fraternities intended to exact a price for my membership. Both contexts offended me and gave weight to my longstanding metaphor of the club, with me standing outside, contemplating my fate as an unwelcome guest.

Chet's membership in the Alpha Phi Alpha fraternity was one of the activities that he liked and in which he participated as a student. He also belonged to the arts association and was an officer in the dormitory and a charter member of the Harvard Key Society. He was a member of the well-known service organization called the Phillips Brooks House, under whose auspices he coached a community basketball team that developed a legendary record of wins over numerous teams. Some of his players did well with their lives, and others ended up in jail. Even with such time-consuming extracurricular activities, however, Chet steadfastly pursued his childhood dream of becoming a doctor. He can't put a finger on where the thought originated, but he recalls with certainty that even people in his hometown knew he intended to be a physician.

Chet spent the summer of 1945 studying Greek at Columbia University summer school, but he's not sure what he did in the summer of 1946. In the summers of 1947 and 1948, however, he worked as a playground instructor in a summer project run by the Lincoln Settlement House in the Bronx. Its director, a Black man named George Gregory, had an innovative idea to combat brawling by youth gangs. Gregory, the first Black basketball captain at Columbia University, hired college athletes to staff the playgrounds; the idea was for the solid college athletes to beat the community youth soundly and persistently in sports. He expected the community youth to respect the collegians eventually, and from there he hoped the youngsters would gradually begin to consider college as a viable pathway for themselves. As a by-product, Gregory expected the gang violence to decrease. Without subjecting the program to serious empirical scrutiny, Chet believes it was an effective initiative.

His own experience in the program made him thoughtful about the future of young Black men who were raised in the midst of so much deprivation and want. He worked in the program alongside a colleague who went on to a distinguished college basketball career until he was disgraced because he was caught shaving points. Another individual played sports for an Ivy League college, continued graduate work at Harvard, and then ultimately got caught in another type of scandal. These vignettes make Chet contemplate how so many Black males waste the rare privileges they are given. He thinks it is hard for individuals who have always had so little of financial and material substance in their lives to resist the temptation of easy money. It's in this sort of discussion one sees the forgiving side of Chet emerge, with the capacity to explain sympathetically the bad things that befall some Blacks.

Chet explains that he occasionally dated Black women from local colleges, although there was no particular person who steadily occupied his time. He also thinks in retrospect that male-female interaction during the collegiate years was less central then than it is now. He describes it as instructive that a White female very familiar to him once denied knowing him when someone sought to introduce them to each other as she joined a group of students who were chatting.

This leads to a revealing associative memory. Chet recalls a White laboratory technician lecturing him one day about how distasteful it was for the Black boxer Jack Johnson to have been prancing around Boston displaying his undue familiarity with White women. Johnson, of course, was the first Black heavyweight champion, who held the title from 1908 to 1915. Apparently, three of his four wives were White, and he was convicted in 1913 of violating the Mann Act. He died in 1946 after being the focus of considerable White hostility, based mostly on his indiscreet and flashy activities with White women. There again was Samuel's preachment about the problematic White fruit. So Chet redoubled his caution but did not cease his entanglements with White women, recalling with some amusement how he met them away from the prying eyes of a Cambridge public unsophisticated in interracial sexual matters.

In response to the question about what difficulties he imagined getting into if his activities had been discovered, Chet concedes that he did not wish to be unpopular, which was the fate that awaited Blacks who trod on this canon that was obviously so sacred to Whites. But his idea of being popular was for people to want him more than he wanted them, a daring way to frame Black-White interactions of the late 1940s in the United States of America. This popularity, this unstable equilibrium, was built on personal charm and clear intellectual and social achievement. Yet, to his mind, it was easily threatened by the basic transgression of being publicly discovered to have been unduly familiar with White women. The whole thing also evoked a certain dissatisfaction because he knew in the social codes of the 1940s that a Black-White relationship could go nowhere, and there was as lucid as ever in his mind the ineffaceable conclusion that a White wife was not an option for him. The eventual connection to a Black spouse was as predictable as the following of the night by intrusion of the daylight sun, welcome or not. Still, Chet observes that he realized White women often found him attractive. Of course, Hettie had done her best to reinforce his sense of being admired by all women, as she constantly told him of those who thought him good-looking. It strikes me, then, that Chet is indeed a very striking physical specimen, with or without his obvious personal charm. You can't miss his imposing height. But there is also the chocolate skin that reminds me of his mother's Native American background, and the gently curling hair, now white, that testifies to a host of mixtures effected in past generations through cross-racial loving. Chet's clearly attractive physique taunts those who rant about racial purity and makes promises to the adventurous. It isn't difficult at all to imagine that women would be curious about what else lies behind the cultured patina.

Previously, Chet and I had discussed the parental advice which counseled him to be cautious with Whites in general and with White women in particular. At this point, he reinforces it with the memory of newspapers in the 1940s carrying headlines about Black men being lynched because of their connection to White women. Furthermore, there was also the popular folklore about White women who used their feminine wiles to seduce Black men and get them into trouble. I can't help making the important observation that this sensitivity about White women, although being a pronounced theme in his early life, never really becomes a sustained theme in his philosophizing about Black-White relationships.

The observation takes us into the more general theme of his pursuing what I like to call a pattern of restricted social interaction with Whites. Chet, for example, accepts few social invitations from White colleagues at Harvard. He even avoids faculty meetings, with the stated rationale of protecting himself from constant microtrauma. He's not even anxious to interact with deans. He explains that from kindergarten through university he's been in predominantly White institutions and has had to find ways of protecting himself. Consequently, he rarely initiates interaction with Whites and in fact promotes distance from them. When he does interact with them, he wants to be in a position of influence, if not ultimately in control. He puts important emphasis on the distinction between being tolerated and being welcomed by Whites. Likewise, it is critical to appreciate the difference between times when Whites act and behave as individuals and when they act and behave as members of a dominant collective. Understanding these essential differences prevents him from ever being disappointed by their unthinking racist behavior. The restricted social interaction also frees him, Chet explains, to contemplate more freely what Blacks should do and how they should behave in a world so thoroughly influenced by racialist thinking. He points out that unrestricted social interaction would not free him to think, for example, about the implications of having Black terrorist groups in operation.

I remain frozen in reflection for a few minutes, and I suddenly realize how independent his thinking truly is and how hard he works to be able to concentrate fully on the interest of Blacks. It reminds me of an observation he has made on several occasions, and which I have repeatedly failed to grasp in its full import. It is that those Whites in power who make policy rarely, if ever, consider the impact that their decisions will have on Blacks. Whites have therefore freed themselves from having to think with sensitivity about the Blacks around them. Chet consequently considers it essential for at least some Black intellectuals to focus on Black interests, and to do so with clarity and sustained commitment—but not off in some separatist environment—right there in the midst of White-controlled institutions. I have yet to grasp all it means when he argues that restricting his social interaction with Whites gives freedom to his intellect. But I suspect that he exerts more control over interactions with White males, which paradoxically ignores Samuel's teaching about White women. I note, too, to myself what it must mean when a Black intellectual as gentle as Chet Pierce reflects on the possibilities of Black terrorist groups. There's a rumbling internal potential for explosiveness that Chet rarely reveals.

All of this leads us full circle to the conclusion that he has never felt welcome at Harvard. I question this assumption with as much vigor as I can muster, and I argue that his achievements belie his opinion: He was an undergraduate and then a graduate student at Harvard; he had a postgraduate Whitehead Fellowship for a year; he was a Marshal and consequently a permanent officer of his senior class; he played on several Harvard varsity teams; he was elected to the Medical School Alumni Council; he has served on three distinct Harvard faculties as a professor; he is even the parent of a Harvard graduate, as his daughter, Diane, graduated from the Harvard Law School. He still claims he has never felt he belonged at Harvard.

Chet goes on to recount another vignette. During his first week at the Medical School, one of his classmates wanted to visit the Business School to see a friend, and Chet agreed to take him there and show him around. At the Business School, Chet got separated from his classmate. But the classmate's friend saw Chet and walked over to him and asked Chet if he belonged there. Chet says he was amazed that a White man, who had been at the Business School only a few days, could be so relaxed as to question someone else about belonging at Harvard. Chet then hastens to add that he doesn't mean to suggest Harvard has nothing to offer him or other Blacks. He can still use an institution like Harvard effectively without really belonging there.

Chet waxes eloquent to prove his thesis. He recalls his perception as a college undergraduate that he had to struggle more than the White students. He also describes his feeling that he could more easily bond with other Black students than with Whites because the Blacks instinctively understood how as a class they would be treated in certain contexts. He tells of the experience while attending High Table in Lowell House when a professor said to him, "You, Black man, where do you come from?" Chet argues that the professor could have addressed him as the man wearing glasses. But the professor intended to be demeaning. Chet drives the point home with the following tale: A fellow student once told him that he knew more English than Chet did. When asked why this was evident, the student replied that the fact spoke for itself. Chet was of course struck by the White student's certainty of his own superior knowledge. He adds, with a flicker of satisfaction, that the student later flunked out of Harvard.

He returns once again to the counsel provided by his parents, who were insistent that Whites generally perceived Blacks as being inferior. In turn, he considers it remarkable when White people treat him well. He proceeds passionately with the argument. Whites retain this presumption of superiority, he asserts, and Blacks should consider it expected thinking from them. Chet garners more proof for his thesis. He once saw a White drunk on the sidewalk trying to shake the hand of every passerby. When Chet reached the drunk, however, the man, even in the depth of his inebriation, sought to avoid shaking hands with him. This is, for Chet, confirmation of his hypothesis.

I just won't let the matter go. I ask him to consider how his life would have been different if his parents had told him nothing about racism. In response, he claims that he would have been less well prepared for the interaction with Whites, and this in turn would have rendered him even more vulnerable. In any event, he asks that I consider the messages coming from other directions, from other sources. For example, on television there is the common scenario of a White person solving a problem with cleverness and effectiveness, whereas the Black individual is seen confronting similar problems with violence or bumbling ineffectiveness. He avers that Blacks are shown to be childlike, needing direction, being incapable; they exist for the entertainment of Whites and are not expected to be in positions of authority and leadership. That is why Blacks in the real world need to be cautious, on their guard, and always prepared to be treated in a demeaning manner that may result in their feeling trivialized.

I point out a possible problem in his argument. Some of our own Black colleagues take his same thesis and then jump to the conclusion that Blacks should simply stay away from places like Harvard. Chet returns to the notion that it is important for Blacks to be aware of how they can use institutions like Harvard. It is also clear he does not advocate all-Black, separatist thinking. I explain my worry that individuals following his view might wear themselves out remaining always on guard against insults from Whites. He agrees it requires technique and experience to protect against being inexorably worn down by the race struggle in this country. I realize that for the time being, I have to let this theme go. But I recognize that I am not satisfied. This business of belonging has long been important to me, and if, with all his credentials and his experience, Chet doesn't feel he belongs at Harvard, what Black person really has a chance of honestly feeling welcome there? Put another way, does Chet see much hope for the future regarding the way Blacks will use White institutions? I know that I have framed the question badly. Chet is making a point that I just won't grasp. He makes a distinction between using an institution and feeling one is a part of it. I see membership as a necessary accompaniment to use. It is clear we see the landscape differently. I know this is at the heart of a more general thesis I have constructed in my head: I am offended by the sense of being simply tolerated at places like Yale (or Harvard or whatever other elite institution one chooses to think about). This is linked to my passionate claim that Blacks genuinely add something valuable to every environment. If we do, then we must not simply make use of Yale; we must assert a genuine belief that we belong there in the same way that any other ethnic or cultural group does.

But to return to the story: Chet decided to apply for admission to the Harvard Medical School. During his undergraduate years he had constantly heard good things about the Medical School and he thought it natural to apply there, although he had also applied elsewhere for training. Harvard was the first institution to accept him, and Harvard it was. Chet completed his undergraduate studies in January 1948 but formally obtained his diploma in June. Between January and September, he had several jobs. First, he worked for David Jones, President of Bennett College, in a position that was related to the United Negro College Fund. It was a fortuitous assignment. Bennett College is located in Greensboro, North Carolina, and it was there that Chet met Jocelyn Patricia Blanchet, who was a senior at the top of her class at Bennett and was considering graduate work in California or New York. By the time he returned North in April, Chet was completely in love. He wrote to her often, and their relationship blossomed. She invited him to return to Bennett for her graduation and to meet her parents. Then they traveled together on a segregated train and returned to Glen Cove, where she met Hettie and successfully courted her future mother-in-law's affections. From there, she accompanied Hettie and Chet to Cambridge for his graduation. Miss Blanchet, whom Chet loves to call Patsy, decided not to go to UCLA for further study and opted instead for graduate work at Columbia University's Teachers College. In the summer, Chet returned to work in the New York City playground.

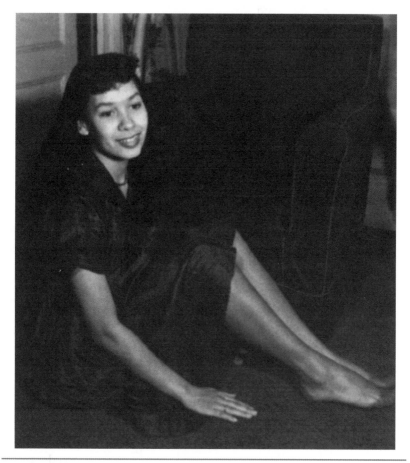

Jocelyn Pierce, 1949.

In the autumn, while strolling on a footbridge across from one of the Harvard Houses, Chet asked Patsy to marry him. At Thanksgiving, the Blanchet family all traveled to Glen Cove, and Chet and Patsy announced their formal engagement. In discussing this marriage proposal, Chet acknowledges having had a profound fear of being rejected, so he did all he could to make sure that Patsy would accept his marriage invitation. Originally, he had never thought he would marry before finishing medical school, but now he was anxious about losing her. This was a fear he had contemplated as a child, the possible rejection as a suitor. I ask whether he had reflected on the origins of this anguish. In response, he reminds me of his general preoccupation as a child with his physical appearance and his envy of brother Burton's lovely curly hair. He talks, too, of his discomfort when associating with the "Black betters," a term once used to describe the children of parents from the Black upper class. And for the first time in our discussion, Chet says he had two left feet, lacked the rhythmic grace of his two brothers, and never danced well at all.

Not surprisingly, of course, Samuel and Hettie loved putting on parties for the three boys and inviting children from the class of "Black betters." Some of these were children Ace had met when he was at Camp Atwater, children of professionals whom Hettie and Samuel felt their own children should rightly get to know. But Chet was not comfortable with these individuals. He had a nagging sense that they came from some sort of superior stock, even though his own parents were easily the economic equal of many of the "betters."

Chet makes the linkage back to his uneasy feeling of being potentially rejected by Patsy. She came from a family with what he describes as "social credentials." Patsy was the daughter of Osceola and Daisy Blanchet, a Black Creole family from New Orleans, and it was apparently well known that Creole families didn't much take to marrying outside their group. Besides, Chet wasn't sure how they would take to his dark skin, and he knew his Harvard diploma wouldn't make much difference to many Creole people. He didn't want to be seen as a hanger-on or a gate crasher. He wanted to be sure he'd be welcomed by Patsy and her family. So by the time he asked for her hand, he was confident of the response.

I am taken by this emerging theme of not belonging, of Chet's discomfort in situations controlled by the dominant White group or by others he thinks are somehow his betters. It is intriguing, too, that he can follow the theme back to what he perceives as its antecedents. Indeed, it is hard to see the obese little boy in the six-foot-four-inch adult, and it is even more difficult to picture the hesitant, fearful child who took so much refuge in his mother's protection in the internationally known Harvard professor who has garnered so many honors. But Chet has no trouble at all in contrasting himself with his cosmopolitan brother, Burton, who associates with a broad spectrum of people and always seems comfortable in any social situation.

In September 1948, with the required microscope in hand and all requisite school fees paid, Chet found his single room in Vanderbilt Hall at the Harvard Medical School. The question of roommates didn't arise in this context, and everybody shared the common bathroom area. The class in the basic science years numbered about 125 students, and in the clinical years it ballooned to about 150 with the influx of transfer students from the 2-year medical schools. In the class of 1952, there were about six women and three Blacks. Chet recalls that the bacteriologist William Augustus Hinton, himself a Harvard Medical School graduate, was the only Black faculty member. Dr. Hinton lectured on syphilis, a subject for which he was recognized as a world-class expert. And by Chet's final year, another Black physician, psychiatrist Frances Bonner, was teaching at Massachusetts General Hospital.

At the end of an uneventful first year, Chet married Patsy in June 1949. The rationale for marriage was a mixture of emotional passion and cool-headed economic reasoning. Patsy and he could make it on their own without anyone else's support, particularly if she worked and they rented a house owned by one of Chet's aunts. Besides, many students in those days were getting married. Patsy had received a teaching offer from Prairie View A&M College in Texas, but she turned it down to become Chet's bride.

Chet says he wanted a very small wedding. However, Hettie had other ideas, and it became a somewhat larger affair. She took control of the planning of a ritual that rightly belonged to the bride's family. As a gesture of compromise to Chet, Hettie allowed the wedding to be held "in the middle of the day, in the middle of the week, in the middle of the month," a time Chet hoped would facilitate the attendance of only a few guests. He and his bride took off for Boston after the ceremony in Glen Cove's Calvary AME Church. There were only a few people from New Orleans, and Francesco Scavullo took the wedding pictures, on strict instructions from the well-organized Hettie. The return to Boston, like the first trip from Bennett College to Glen Cove, was by train; this means of travel has taken on special meaning for Chet over the years. Hettie also ordered the ring for Patsy, and for Chet, she provided the ring she had saved from the deceased Samuel. I had to comment on the fact that Hettie had not given the ring to Ace, who had married about a year before Chet did. There is no immediate answer forthcoming, but then I prod him with the observation that Hettie had saved the ring for her "Baby Boy." He responds with his view that he can say little about Hettie's motivations regarding the gift of the ring. But he concedes that of the three boys, he had stayed closest to their mother during his childhood years, and he had probably been the child she found most responsive to her influence.

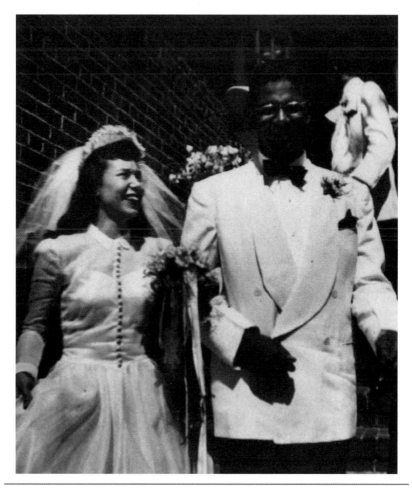

Chester and Jocelyn Pierce on their wedding day, June 15, 1949.

The summer of 1949 brought harsh reality that diluted the romantic feelings somewhat. Patsy, even with a master's degree from Columbia, found it hard to get work, although she eventually was hired by the personnel department of the Massachusetts Institute of Technology, in a position Chet feels was significantly below what her education had prepared her for. He had made his decision to marry when he did partly because he'd been promised the financial security of a summer job working on a railroad. However, when he showed up to claim the work, the promise simply evaporated. Wishing to stay independent and self-reliant, he took what he could get and even worked a few weeks as a stevedore and a furniture mover. In some desperation, he sought the help of an employment office and was offered a job washing walls and floors at the Massachusetts General Hospital. As fate would have it, a classmate came by one day to see him and found him on his knees scrubbing a floor. Chet hasn't forgotten the irony in his having to scrub floors while his White classmates had jobs in laboratories. That experience around employment was in a way similar to the feeling evoked by his walking onto a hospital ward wearing the medical students' traditional white coat only to be asked if he was the barber.

Chet reports that he blossomed in the clinical years, despite the somewhat tentative beginning. He gained confidence and felt he could do well, even though he acknowledges that he felt some distance from the students who were academically at the top of the class. But he still concluded that patients and teachers liked him. In his junior year, for example, he was admitted to the Boylston Society, which was open only to upperclassmen. The group met once a month, and a student usually presented a paper at dinner. In his senior year, Chet presented work on the Plague of Athens in which he explored how major disasters like plagues influenced human behavior. Incidentally, Dr. John Enders, who later won the Nobel Prize in Medicine, was the faculty discussant of that paper. In spite of Chet's lifelong ambition to be a pediatrician, the recognition by teachers of his skills in psychiatry helped nudge him along the road to changing his mind about his specialty. His interest in psychiatry led to a discussion with Frances Bonner, a Black female psychoanalyst at Mass General, who recommended that he go to the University of Cincinnati for psychiatric training. He was already being attracted by the apparent limitlessness of psychiatry and its open breadth and adaptability to physicians with unusual interests. Patsy did not interfere with or attempt to influence his specialty choice. She also never pushed him in any particular direction so that he would make money. He's sure that in medical school he did not consider the possibility of an academic career, and he had no special confidence that he would even make a comfortable living in psychiatry. He was certainly not sure that any White person would pay to see a Black psychiatrist, nor did he believe there were numerous Blacks possessed of sufficient resources to support a Black psychiatrist in private practice. But with his love at his side, he took off for the University of Cincinnati to start his rotating internship and his training in psychiatry without even attending his own medical school graduation in June 1952.

In adhering to his penchant for doing things in sharp sequence, Chet went directly to medical school after completing his undergraduate degree. I, on the other hand, served in the U.S. Army after Harvard and did a stint in Vietnam. Military service was particularly instructive, as I learned so well that Black skin was not always the best adhesive for as-suring solid brotherhood. My Black sergeant reminded me periodically that he was not my brother. The lessons were expensive but worth learning. Still, I was glad when my 2 years had passed and I could walk the streets as a civilian. I eventually went to France to study medicine and found there a wonderfully different ambience.

The French culture and new friends brought me to life again after the amazing experience of war. But even France and love have never to-tally effaced the grindingly oppressive inner feelings evoked when I contemplate the American political authorities sitting at their desks and authorizing that more bombs be dropped. They also made it clear that their bombs had more moral authority than the North Vietnamese bombs. Because I studied at the University of Strasbourg, I had ample opportunities to talk to Alsatians about war—what it did to human be-ings, and the mythical claim that in war one nation is more humane than another.

France also afforded me the chance to explore another brand of co-lonialism and to reflect on the French attitude toward citizens of coun-tries like Algeria and Morocco. I struggled with the writings of Fanon just as much as I devoured the poems of Apollinaire and the sculptures of Rodin. I spent long hours interviewing patients who were immigrant workers in France. I was fascinated by my impression that their hand injuries took longer to heal than similar hand trauma in my White French patients. I wanted to know why. My preoccupation with the psy-chosocial terrain that could lead to different healing times between French and North African workers afflicted with similar surgical trauma had me well on my way to becoming a psychiatrist before I re-alized it.

3

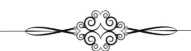

The Cincinnati and Navy Years

The internship year for most physicians is typically very hectic, and for Chester Pierce it was no different. He and Patsy, with the help of a Black Episcopal pastor, found a one-room efficiency apartment in the Black section of Cincinnati. He made the princely sum of $15 a month, which was just about enough to buy the ice cream Patsy loved so much. She worked as a librarian, finally using the skills learned in her college major of library science. The social events were less frequent than they had grown accustomed to in Boston, but their circle of friends gradually expanded with the passage of time.

They attended a Methodist church that was conveniently located in the neighborhood. Opting for Methodism might have represented a good family compromise, given Chet's AME background and Patsy's long connection to the Congregational Church. By his internship year, Chet had settled, to his own satisfaction, any arguments with himself over God and about the importance of supporting the Black church as an important community institution. He believed earnestly that there was a God and felt God's existence was readily confirmed by his experiences in medical school. But he was less confident about this business of Jesus having been the son of God. He acknowledged the existence of the Master as a historical figure and noted that Tacitus, the Roman historian, had mentioned Jesus in his writings. But the existence of a filial connection between Jesus and God didn't quite ring true in Chet's analysis.

I easily follow Chet's thinking here and realize that he has neatly framed one of the important dilemmas in my own life. This internal human need for a belief in God can be overwhelmingly powerful, and I recall that it hit me, too, like a sledgehammer when I was in medical school. It must have been the experience of confronting the marvelously poetic structure and function of the human body, coupled with the often utter helplessness of physicians facing the relentless progression of disease and degenerative processes. But I know that the medical school years were also a time in my life when I needed God and felt He was there. In spite of that very personal reality, like Chet, I cannot be persuaded of certain notions that some Christian churches hold so very dear. I reject, with no regret at all, the ludicrous idea that men alone can be priests because their gender is so superior to that of women. Recently, my brother asked me how I can so readily afford to dispense with logic in talking about my need for God, then lean so heavily on it when I talk about the issue of elevating women to the priesthood. I had no answer for him. I have just never found it easy to follow my preacher-father's recommendation that one should just suspend all reasoning faculties when dealing with God and religion. For him it was so clear: If you believed in the Lord Jesus Christ, everything else would fall into place. So I was with Chet on this one, even if our stance was sometimes logical and other times devoid of logic.

One thing he had absolutely no doubts about was his new wife. Patsy was obviously a special presence in Chet's life, and he enjoyed their life together, with special touches such as her greeting him after work with a bath already drawn. He had read articles about the importance of not waiting too late in marriage to start a family, so he and Patsy decided to take the plunge. She quickly became pregnant, and they were delighted with the arrival of Diane Blanchet Pierce on August 26, 1953. Chet went home to Glen Cove to consult with a banker and ended up with his first loan—totaling $4,000—because he wanted to be sure to have enough money to support his enlarged family, particularly since Patsy wouldn't be returning to work. There was even enough money to buy a used car. These events made for a speedy passage of the internship year. However, in spite of the outstanding performance in surgery that prompted invitations for him to enter surgical training, in 1953 Chet began his specialty training in psychiatry, still not clear about where his career plans were ultimately headed.

One memory from the internship year still stands out clearly for Chet. At about one o'clock in the morning, Chet was working in a little clinical laboratory that used to be a commonplace structure on hospital services. It was where interns routinely performed studies on patients' urine and blood, for example. Some patients could see into that particular laboratory directly from their beds on the unit. A White female patient called to Chet from her bed, and he responded that he would drop by to see her a little later because right then he was busy. She told him to come immediately or she would shout that he was trying to rape her. Because he was unsure of what she would do, he went over to talk to her. He explained to me that she only wanted attention, with no sexual implications, even though he recalled her being somewhat flirtatious. His memory about any other details of the interaction isn't clear, but he knew she was putting him in a bind. To this day, he has not forgotten the sensation of being manipulated in such a blatantly racist manner. Recall that at the time of the incident Samuel's lectures weren't that far distant. Of course, the White woman's threat is every Black physician's nightmare and the proverbial razor held to every Black man's throat. I remain puzzled by the apparent nonchalance with which he recounts that whole tale. In pleasant contrast, Chet stated that in the same internship year, a Black woman, in appreciation of his clinical interaction with her, named her newborn baby after him.

At lunch the same day Chet told me about the incident with the White female patient, our conversation turned to the subject of how such negative experiences have a cumulative impact. As he sees it, the repetitive traumatic interactions batter Blacks into being conservative in their thinking and very cautious in their creative initiatives by making them worry consistently about not losing what they have. The experiences have the effect of making them fall short of ever feeling that they are "to the manor born." Of course, it is another way of explaining Blacks' sense of not belonging. Chet doesn't push the point, and I let it drop with him. But I go on thinking to myself that although a number of Blacks are battered into conservatism, many others are simply beaten into submission. These unlucky individuals give up and minimize their interactions with the White world, preferring to seek their whole future in the Black community.

In the 1953–1954 academic year, Chet and his family moved into an attic apartment to minimize expenses. He began his first foray into teaching by lecturing to nurses on psychopathology. He also recalled a growing interest in Alzheimer's disease and its treatment with vitamins.

Around this time, Meharry Medical College officials got wind of the fact that Chet was taking psychiatric training at the University of Cincinnati and sent a professor of medicine to invite him to visit their school. Chet was preparing for the visit when Maurice Levine, head of Cincinnati's Department of Psychiatry, told Chester not to rush into any decisions about his career because Levine was considering him for future faculty status. Chet maintains this all came as a surprise to him, and he had never even seriously considered academic life as a career. Still, he made the visit to Meharry, and school officials offered to finance the rest of his residency training at Cincinnati if he would promise to join the Meharry faculty for at least 1 year when his training was completed. Although the Meharry offer was tempting, Chet turned it down because he ultimately concluded that there would be chances for other offers.

Although Chet doesn't verbalize it directly, I recognize the difficult choice that faces Black professionals when they have to decide between joining a historically Black institution and remaining with a predominantly White one. The discussion even evoked my own struggle, years ago, over joining Yale or staying at an urban facility in New York, delivering service primarily to minority group members. I remember the struggle well because more than one Black friend or colleague had brazenly accused me of selling out when I finally announced I was leaving New York to join the Yale faculty. My militant friends weren't much impressed by the argument that Blacks can play different roles in the struggle on behalf of the larger group. They thought the situation was straightforwardly simple. Black professionals who join places like Yale are inherently renouncing their solemn duty and role. Furthermore, such professionals are inexorably transformed by the White institution and ultimately turn their backs on their Black brothers and sisters. Although it may be a legitimate point of view, I will not concede the point. Furthermore, I thought then—and still do now—that it must be awful tyranny if all Black professionals are to be confined to service in Black institutions. I base my position first on the cardinal principle that Black people must work hard to safeguard their individual autonomy, even against incursions from other Blacks. The second major principle I add is that just because Black professionals work in a predominantly White institution, this does not mean they have renounced their ethnic identities or commitments to the struggle on behalf of the larger ethnic group. Such a claim maligns Black professionals who have opted to work outside predominantly Black organizations.

In any event, the question of how to contend with the difficult problem of the interaction between the dominant White group and the non-dominant Black group in the United States cannot be resolved simply by requiring all the Black talent to reject any role at all in the White group and to keep their activities circumscribed within the Black group. Such a requirement, of course, would have kept Chet Pierce on a very limited course. As we shall see, I think Chet participated substantially in White institutions while still keeping a powerful presence in the struggle on behalf of Black Americans. And while he was in Cincinnati, two older professional couples, the Spencers and the Houghs, helped Chet in this endeavor.

Chet's worrying over the Meharry dilemma was temporarily shelved because of the impact of the doctors' military draft. In 1954, he was ordered to report to the U.S. Navy, even though he'd expressed a clear interest in the Air Force. Then he wished for assignment to an aircraft carrier and exposure to flight training, hoping eventually to become a flight surgeon. But none of these hopes materialized. His civilian boss had recommended him highly, and Chet was assigned to be a psychiatrist at the Great Lakes Naval Base. He explains, with his usual equanimity, that he had expected a bad assignment and he got it. He ended up in a training unit doing screening assessments of all kinds of trainees, a job that carried less glamour and prestige than the coveted assignments to the base hospital, for example. With an interesting mixture of bitterness and smugness, Chet notes that a White medical school classmate mobilized at the same time was assigned to the hospital. There is bitterness because he is persuaded that the difference in assignments was based on race; the smugness comes from his recognition that despite the bad assignment, it turned out to be one of the best things that ever happened to him.

As has occurred so many other times in Chet's life, this bad placement became even pleasant and worthwhile because of a fortuitous convergence of elements. First, his particular assignment ultimately left him lots of free time that he used profitably to read all manner of textbooks and articles. Then the other psychiatrists in the unit, all more experienced than he, took a serious hand in his supervision and made sure that he treated a wide variety of patients. The result was that the American Board of Psychiatry and Neurology (ABPN) translated his 2 military years into academic credit: 1 year of didactic training and 1 year of practical experience. In those days, the ABPN required 3 years of didactic training and 2 years of practical experience before one could take the specialty examination.

Chet's commanding officer was also immensely supportive. Chet even recalled how this officer personally accompanied him as Chet bought his first officer's uniform. Chet also talked fondly of Jim Stuart, a White medical corpsman who was profoundly helpful and who later went on to medical school and became a psychiatrist. The assignment additionally permitted Chet access to enlisted men who could perform tasks for him such as transporting numerous heavy books to and from the base library. With all the free time available, Chet volunteered to take other colleagues' assignments in running clinics. He particularly enjoyed covering the mandatory general medical clinics, a task that understandably made anxious his older colleagues who had left general medicine a few years back. The free time allowed his participation in sports, especially basketball. With the tacit support of his supportive commanding officer, he fraternized with enlisted men and played competitive sports with them. His colleagues advised him to spend time gaining clinical experience working at the base's brig, the military prison, and he did it energetically.

Chet loved taking medical watch at the base's infirmary and enjoyed keeping his skills honed in general medicine. He acknowledges, too, that he had youth and energy, never felt exploited, and appreciated how much his older colleagues gave him in supervision and advice. For example, one of them advised him which professional associations to join and then proceeded to sponsor Chet for membership. Even in the clinical time he spent at the base prison, he was lucky to make special contacts. There he met the marine colonel in charge of the brig, who invited him to join his weekly commander's rounds when he would review all the prisoners who were being held in detention. The colonel taught Chet a lot about human beings and allowed him to be present when the colonel conducted his special weekly office hours during which prisoners were allowed to speak to the colonel.

I note here how helpful to Chet so many Whites were during these military years, and it will certainly come up at other phases in his development. In fact, it has also been a recurrent theme in my own maturing. At key points in my life, Whites have been simply generous and helpful. Many of those who have had a significant influence on my life have been Jews. I assume it was mere coincidence. But I still remember in the short period I spent at Brooklyn's Boys High School that it was a Jewish teacher who had me transfer from the regular academic track to the special scholarship track. From then on, two Jewish female grade advisors took me under their maternal wings and had me headed for Harvard before I could even reflect on all the implications of such a decision. That was just the beginning of a string of Jewish helpers who would appear at crucial moments in my life and keep me balanced and on track.

One central task that Chet performed was to screen all naval trainees before they began basic training, concentrating on the question of whether the trainee was likely to complete his training successfully. It was in the midst of performing such screening that Chet encountered the serious military problem of enuresis, better known as bedwetting. This was a practical problem for the Navy, and the official policy was that individuals who wet their beds should be discharged because it was thought they could potentially create substantial morale problems and ultimately compromise the mission of the organization. Such persons were seen as not representing the Navy's view of the symbolic macho warrior. In addition, there was concern that in a situation where bunks were closely placed one on top of the other, the seaman in the bottom bunk would be patently offended by urine seeping through on him from above. There might also be unpleasant odors that developed as a result of dried urine in the bedding. Commanders certainly thought that unit personnel might tease an identified individual who wet his bed or even harass him physically.

The screening procedures were therefore intended to bring to the attention of the command structure those individuals with all sorts of troubling histories, including bedwetting. The objective was to separate these servicemen from the Navy. Chet Pierce was intrigued by the obvious significance of the enuresis problem in the context of naval and general military efficiency and organization. I wonder whether he was attracted by the idea that the affected seamen were a group of individuals who were really excluded from the overall organization and, in a psychological sense, did not belong in the Navy—or rather, they did not belong to the Navy. The military organization ultimately labeled them and turned them into outsiders. It is ironic, then, that Chet, who would continue throughout his life to contend with the problem of belonging to White-dominated organizations such as Harvard, saw an opportunity to engage in a systematic study of another group that defined the phenomenon of nonbelonging.

It is evident that it helped to have ready access to large numbers of people who could easily provide Chet a population for the study of the bedwetting disorder. He therefore considered what might be important to learn about individuals who wet their beds. The first issue was to confirm the diagnosis of bedwetting because everybody knew that malingering was not unknown among youngsters seeking to get free of military service. This particular problem was solved to a significant degree by having social service organizations confirm the diagnosis through interviews with the seamen's relatives and family physicians. The second task was to explore the relationships between the seamen and important others in their lives and to paint a psychodynamic picture of the individual bedwetter.

Chet also theorized that there might be something unique about the brain activity of individuals who wet their beds, and he concluded that an electroencephalogram (EEG) might provide the essential information about brain function, together with extensive psychological testing. Chet was not a psychologist, and he was also not trained in reading EEGs. So he contacted Captain H. H. Lipcon, a physician board-certified in both psychiatry and neurology, who was the one who generally interpreted EEGs on Chet's base. Lipcon not only agreed to teach Chet how to read the brain tracings but also became an enthusiastic participant in the studies. Lieutenant Howard Noble, a combat-decorated executive officer of Chet's unit and a psychologist, also agreed to provide expertise that was necessary for the successful completion of the work. As Chet found out, Lipcon and Noble were good friends, which not only made the practical aspects of the work easier to implement but also ensured that they would become his solid supporters. This was important because he needed their help to find his way through the political terrain that is so often a part of research field studies with large experimental groups. In another attempt to facilitate navigation of the political waters, Chet sought and received approval from the base commander for the studies he was contemplating. It turned out the base commander had been a member of a military team that had played football against Harvard some years earlier, and he remembered Chet quite well. This memorable piece of luck resulted in Chet's obtaining a building where he could house the recruits he was investigating and also perform EEGs and other studies.

Chet's work on what he called the common problem of symptomatic immaturity habits is indeed an interesting historical note in the annals of military psychiatry. That bedwetting should have been considered such an important issue at the time, significant enough to require the separation of those with enuresis from military service, seems hard to understand now. But in the context of the 1950s, Chet and his colleagues recognized the considerable potential for economic and morale problems the Navy faced as a result of seamen with enuresis. It was expected that these individuals would have substantial difficulty in completing basic training, and even after discharge from the Navy, would not reintegrate easily into civilian life. One out of every hundred men entering naval service at the Great Lakes base was discharged because of enuresis, and this occurred prior to completion of basic training.

Chet and his colleagues therefore set about to carry out clinical, laboratory, and electroencephalographic studies of bedwetting. The intent was to accumulate enough information on those affected to facilitate eventual determination of which recruits might be rehabilitated for continued naval duty and which ones could not be rehabilitated and therefore should be quickly separated from the service. In short, was there a sound rationale for excluding these young men from military service and then making dire predictions about their future capacity to adapt to civilian life?

The experimental group was composed of 120 recruits equally divided into two groups, with and without enuresis. The researchers acknowledged that the control and experimental groups were not closely matched. However, the control group of Electronics School students was considered by the Navy to represent individuals who were highly suitable for military service, in contrast to individuals with the disorder, who were labeled as unsuitable. Twenty-five percent of the recruits with the disorder had abnormal EEGs, in contrast to a single control group member. Interestingly, that group member had suffered from enuresis until he was 15 years old and also had a positive family history of enuresis. Seventy-five percent of the experimental group had a positive family history of enuresis, in contrast to 17% of the control subjects. The experimental group described 76 genitourinary complaints in comparison to 4 complaints from the control group. These complaints focused on matters such as urinary urgency, frequent urination, and pain or burning on urination. Seventy-three percent of the experimental group volunteered feelings of shame and embarrassment over their bedwetting, and they showed substantially more dependency traits than did the control group. There was also more chronic illness in the parents of experimental group members than among control group members.

These findings caused Chet's group to ponder the implications. The preponderance of the positive EEGs among members of the experimental group and their very strong family history of enuresis suggested that there was some biological factor that accounted for the disorder. The researchers also wondered whether the biological disturbance, whatever it was, might in a more general way be responsible for sleep disturbances in the affected individuals. One particular sleep disturbance that interested them was somnambulism, or sleepwalking, a condition that had special importance to any naval command interested in minimizing accidents aboard ship. Chet and his colleagues confirmed that a significantly large number of their recruits with enuresis were sleepwalkers. They were also shown to have a statistically pertinent past history of epilepsy. So, theoretically, epilepsy, enuresis, and somnambulism could represent different manifestations of some similar biological problem. Not unexpectedly, the biological thesis did not explain all their findings. For instance, it did not shed light on the apparent preoccupation that affected individuals had with genitourinary complaints, nor did the biological theory explain their tendency to be characterologically dependent. Although Chet was also transitorily intrigued by other difficulties that seemed to impair the general performance of Navy recruits—such as poor dentition and stuttering—he was clearly primarily interested in the difficulties that seemed linked to disturbances of sleep. Without recognizing it at first, he was on the way to becoming an expert in the emerging arena of sleep pathophysiology. This area of work would be enhanced through his collaboration with other colleagues once he returned to Cincinnati. For the time being, however, the research results on bedwetting provided some interesting avenues for further exploration but no definitive data on which to base clear policy changes.

In retrospect, Chet concedes that the assignment, which he is confident was intended to be punitive, left him lots of extra time that he used profitably. He is proud of the great breadth of clinical material he observed. He also read psychiatry textbooks cover to cover and took voluminous notes, while making thoughtful use of assistance from a number of White males who simply decided to take him under their wing. Among them were his immediate boss, Commander Albert Zuska, who Chet thinks was a wonderful human being and one of the most brilliant people he has ever met; Captain H.H. Lipcon, the EEG teacher and a sponsor for medical association memberships; and Lieutenant Noble, a psychologist-collaborator on the studies. These connections were invaluable and led to other contacts that stretched on for years after Chet left the Navy. He is also insistent that at the time he had enormous youth and energy; he never felt exploited by the officers in his unit, who were all his senior; and the officers repaid him with substantive advice and supervision. He adds that a recent invitation to consider a job offer was extended to him because of these contacts, as were opportunities over the years to be a consultant to all three branches of the armed forces. It was also with the encouragement of Lipcon and Lieutenant Commander Alan Robertson that Chet undertook to work at the brig and to develop the particular area of forensic psychiatry that would probably be better known today as military prison psychiatry. Chet wrote several descriptive articles that outlined aspects of his work in the brig, including one on the use of brief group therapy with the guards aimed at helping them decrease their general anxiety and improve their performance in handling the detainees. Most of the seamen and marines who were in the brig were being held on AWOL charges, and most of them ultimately had very problematic military careers, even those who had been distinguished in combat. Parenthetically, Chet notes that most people in the brig were White, reflecting directly their proportion in the population in military service at the time.

Chet is positive and zealous in the description of his Navy years. I ascribe a part of his enthusiasm to the fact that he was a physician and was drafted for duty as an officer. In addition, he served his tour of duty stateside and could indulge his passion for intellectual inquiry. I was drafted to be an enlisted man and spent part of my 2 years in South Vietnam. It was 1965 when I first walked through downtown Saigon (now called Ho Chi Minh City) and started making connections to Vietnamese people—and encountered a former classmate of mine from Harvard! I quickly wrote a note back to a friend still at Fort Sam Houston commenting on the obvious disarray of the American troops and commenting on the obvious: that no one in the military understood why we were in Vietnam. My friend showed the missive to an officer, who commented that something ought to be shoved up my backside. I learned then to keep my comments to myself and went on to construct some semblance of a humane existence among nonmilitary Americans and Vietnamese in Saigon. I hated most the military's clear lack of respect for enlisted men in general and privates in particular. But what grated most was the Black sergeant in my unit who sought every occasion to humiliate me and another Black West Indian (who everyone knew had an IQ that bordered on the genius). The military taught me that not all Blacks are my brothers, a lesson I would never forget. Indeed, that sergeant singlehandedly blocked the promotion of the two Blacks in his unit while the White major looked on with a contemptuous smirk. When the other West Indian threatened to complain to the inspector general, the major told him to go ahead, adding that a private's words were not likely to be more persuasive than a major's. But I looked into the major's eyes and saw his contempt and knew he meant that this time his hands were clean. It was the Black sergeant who was oppressing us. When Blacks press other Blacks down, it should not be blamed on White bystanders. Chet's military experience wasn't mine. I came out of the Army with enough anger to last a lifetime, and that is without even contemplating my feelings about how White Americans generally treated the darker-skinned Vietnamese.

It was also during his period of naval service that Chet became interested in sports medicine. The interest was nourished by his friendship with Howard Noble and Jim Stuart, a former college football star. Their discussions led them to ask what information they would need to make predictions about the performance of football players. For example, could a player's performance be predicted by the elements of running speed, lateral reaction time, leg strength, and other variables such as playing experience and psychological preparation? The research team got some technical help from Allan Ryan, who later was the founding editor of *The Physician and Sportsmedicine*. At the time, Ryan was a physician and sports medicine researcher at the University of Wisconsin. They also received permission to try out some of their techniques on the Chicago Cardinals of the National Football League and to use the players as a control group in the study. Although they completed the project, its most problematic aspect remained the experience variable. The study results were never published because certain of the psychological tests were not completed. Still, Chet sees the whole experience as important in sustaining the development of his interest in sports medicine. He recalls with considerable satisfaction the tentative conclusions of the study, which centered on predicting who among the 100 Navy tryouts appearing for the team in August would constitute the top 22 players on the team in November. The researchers actually predicted the top players, including one surprise Black athlete who hadn't played much serious football before.

Chet notes that the question of longer-term prediction was also crucial in the enuresis study, but the Navy at the time would not allow the recruits with enuresis to stay in the service. He also points out that he was a consultant to the study group that later designed a long-term project that persuaded the Navy it could change its policy regarding the seamen with enuresis.

There is one other aspect of his Navy work that Chet talks about with more than a modicum of passion. His unit of psychiatrists and psychologists, under the leadership of Commander Zuska, screened individuals volunteering for hazardous duty, such as service with the divers, in submarines, and in the Antarctic. This particular work helped him to understand how the Navy conceptualized the task of predicting whether an individual would do well in a specialized and stressful context. When I ask about the Antarctic and straightforwardly confess my ignorance about its location and military significance, Chet smilingly indulges me and demonstrates his long-accumulated knowledge about a variety of extreme environments. He points out that the Antarctic is the region at the bottom of the globe, characterized by being the coldest, driest, windiest, and highest continent. Although there are seals, whales, penguins, and birds living in the region, humans do not live there indigenously. When people go there, they must take with them everything they need. The Navy has long had an interest in the region, and the military services have generally influenced the science projects that have been done there. But without saying more, Chet suggests quietly that science is often used as a sort of varnish to cover the real political interests in such regions as the Antarctic. He concludes by noting that 1956 was declared the International Geophysical Year, and many countries had expressed an intention of setting up scientific projects in Antarctica.

In reflecting on some of the things Chet has told me about his tour of duty in the Navy, I raise the question of what pushed him so powerfully to be academically productive. After all, I say, the Navy was not my ideal think tank, and the other naval officers around him were not academics. So what was the source of energy driving the academic scholarship? The central theme of his response is the profound independence the Navy offered him, in addition to the time he had to read and formulate research questions. It was also tremendously helpful to have superiors who genuinely cared about his opinions and views and supported his quest for knowledge. Chet doesn't hesitate to contrast the Navy experience with the large number of individuals he had met in hospitals who were imprecise in using medical and psychiatric jargon. This irritated him, especially when he returned to the residency program, because he had developed the habit of buttressing his thinking with a solid mastery of the technical literature.

I go back to his Navy research on bedwetting, and I point out to Chet that the work evoked some fundamental questions, under the rubric of dependency, about the experimental group's connections to their fathers and mothers. Wishing to probe his own parental linkages some more, I ask once again about the ring Hettie provided for his wedding. This time he provides greater clarity and replies that he wanted a double-ring ceremony but Ace didn't. Without any prodding, he goes on to explain his view that he was probably the favorite child of both his parents and likely, too, among his aunts and cousins.

Unabashedly, I ask what he thinks justifies his being the preferred one, so to speak. He certainly thinks he is more approachable than Ace, and while conceding Burton's great affable character, Chet wonders whether he was always more dependable and compliant than Burton as a child. But while I admit it is easy to see Chet's sensitivity to people, I tell him I don't think one would easily classify him as gregarious. He concedes it and agrees he finds it difficult to initiate contact with people. Especially in early life, he found it hard to say bad things about people and often just remained silent.

I return to Hettie and the theme of dependency. Chet feels she wanted him to go off and be on his own, to make his own life. Before his death, Samuel had also talked that way, promoting the independence of his male children. Chet then adds that Patsy also shared this view, that in a sense, once they left home, "we had no parents." This, he explains, was not meant to deny their parents but more to confirm their independence and the fact that they were accountable to themselves. It is certainly worth noting, too, that by 1956, Chet's last year on active duty, Hettie was already in a sanatorium for treatment of tuberculosis and therefore in no position to assert her views as she had done in the past. Chet can only say that by then he had already lost two other family members to tuberculosis, so he felt a certain psychological immunity to the stigma of TB. He concedes it was bad fortune for her to have caught the disease but also points out that as an intern he had seen lots of TB, which I take as an indication that he had no undue fear of the illness.

I fail to provoke more of an emotional rise from Chet. It makes me reflect on my own behavior when my mother was given the diagnosis of breast cancer and then was subjected to the horrors of a radical mastectomy. I was away in college at the time, but I vaguely recall the sensation of total helplessness, the recognition that there was nothing I could do. Worse, I noted from time to time over the succeeding years her struggles with an artificial breast that just never fit properly and an arm that stayed permanently swollen. But I was never confident enough to ask my mother how much of a burden it was to put up with a diagnosis that raised the specter of death, while also coping with the type of mutilating surgery that only a man could have inflicted on a woman. I held my tongue and have regretted it ever since I became conscious of my silence. I can only guess at Chet's unspoken correspondence with Hettie.

As a transition, I return to Chet's interest in sleep studies and I ask him what his own sleep pattern was like, particularly in those early days. He observes that critical hours of sleep for him were from three to six o'clock in the morning. If he slept from midnight to four, for instance, it wouldn't have the same effect. He also thinks that during his college days he didn't seem to need as much sleep as most people around him, and for most of his life he had slept only 4 hours a night. Things changed somewhat as he reached his late fifties and developed trouble with his prostate. He then had to get up several times a night, which led to more hours being spent in bed, albeit with no corresponding increase in a sense of restfulness. He notes, too, that at one time he could sleep any time he wanted and also wake up at will. But such dominance of his sleep pattern progressively eluded him with passing years. Chet makes one further point about the distinction between macro and micro working hours. He often tried to do lots of work between Monday and Wednesday, thereby allowing himself the rest of the week to travel and do other things. That permitted him the chance to compensate correspondingly with the necessary hours of sleep.

I pass then to what I have come to identify as an episode with the potential to be a marker event in Chet Pierce's life. It must have been around 1956 when the famous Adam Clayton Powell Jr., suggested in a speech that all the Blacks in the country should collectively bring the economy to a halt by staying away from work. Chet agreed to participate in this call to arms and worked it out with three Black enlisted men not to report for duty. Chet could not recall any major discussion about planning to take this step. He just thought it a good thing to do because he recognized that it would dramatically demonstrate the importance of Blacks to the national economy. He could recall no particular objections from Patsy; in addition, there were no racial problems in his unit that could conceivably have helped to catalyze his decision to heed Powell's invitation.

However, he did have to contend with Zuska's superior, the captain who had overall authority over the outfit and to whom Chet had made the traditionally required courtesy visit when he first reported to the base. Chet recalls with a certain bitterness that as soon as he met the officer he knew the man would start to talk about slaves. No sooner thought then it happened. This Southern officer and gentleman quickly started telling Chet that his family had kept a number of slaves, noting also that his brother-in-law was then a U.S. Senator from South Carolina. Chet adds that this same officer was rumored to have once said that his leadership was burdened by having as officers "niggers, Jews, and a Chinaman."

The captain had his own view of Chet's response to Congressman Powell's plan, and he let it be known that he intended to court-martial Chet on several counts: incitement to riot, conduct unbecoming an officer, and contravening the oath of an officer. Fortunately for Chet, Zuska and Noble intervened and persuaded the captain to drop his plans for retribution. So the potentially celebrated affair passed.

I ask Chet how he could have possibly imagined he could get away with it. After all, that was 1955 or 1956, and heroic, revolutionary Black men weren't surviving very well. I additionally point out to Chet that there was other evidence of his provocative behavior, such as his socializing with Jim Stuart, who at the time was a White enlisted man, and his playing sports with enlisted men. Chet agrees that his deportment was problematic and wonders whether he got away with it because in the eyes of many people he was simply an "old jock." But he insists he never intended to make a big splash or a major political statement. It was the right thing to do, and he did it. It was only later that he reflected on the implications, the risk of acting; later on still, he understood better the concept of consequences. I let it pass for the time being. But I mull over my realization that Chet was familiar with many of the reasons people ended up in the brig and I make a mental note to myself to keep my eye on this notion of Chet as a quiet revolutionary and to watch for points where his actions could have cost him dearly, areas where he might have sacrificed a lot for a principle. It is also striking that there was no struggle with Patsy over this. I have great faith in the wives of principled men, and I suspect she blanched at the realization that her husband could have been in the brig while she raised her young family all alone. Too many wives and mothers have taught me that political principles don't raise children and that they don't purchase much at the neighborhood grocery store.

This is not to say that the men and their wives necessarily disagree about the action to be taken. But in my experience, they differ in the way they carry out their assessment of the consequences. Men often keep their eyes on the broad impact of their principled behavior. Their wives remain sensitive to what it all means for them and for the lives of their children. Of course, I did no assessment at all of potential consequences when the Black sergeant came toward me one day and asked where I'd been. Fed up with his repeated wish to hassle me, I stayed silent and quietly stared at him. In military parlance, it was belligerent insubordination. In my own terms, I was struggling to refrain from saying something that would have been overt proof of my insolence and that would have been used against me. The sergeant saw it all as my mocking him. Perhaps he was right. I know it was the lesser of two evils and that I would cope with the consequences, which turned out to be my kissing goodbye any hope of being promoted. In military tradition at the time, this was significant because promotions came easily to those serving in Vietnam.

Chet's 2-year tour of active duty eventually came to an end, and because he was a reservist, he had never seriously considered staying in the Navy. However, he had contemplated extending his stay when it seemed possible that he might go to an assignment in Japan with Commander Zuska. That fell through when Zuska had an accident. Patsy, on the other hand, liked the Navy life, with its amenities and regular work hours, and probably also the prestige of being an officer's wife. Although friends certainly urged him to become a regular Navy officer and give up his reserve status, Chet wasn't sure there was much of a future for a Black military professional. So he left the Navy in 1956 with the rank of lieutenant to finish his residency training at Cincinnati and then spent 3 more years on the faculty there.

Going back to this reduced status was difficult, and Chet concedes readily that he had an inflated idea of his knowledge base but also had the personal arrogance and impatience to get on with his career. As he saw it, after having admirals and Navy captains listen to him and take him seriously, it was hard to be a trainee again. Having no other option, however, he buckled down to complete the remaining training year. Because of his sustained interest in general medicine, Chet had the idea of going to London to study neurology and started to investigate the possibility of doing so. Executing the idea would have required him to save money, and he thought of working in a nearby state hospital to make the extra income. The department head, Maurice Levine, nixed both the London and the state hospital ideas and instead proposed that Chet apply to the National Institute of Mental Health (NIMH) for a Career Teacher Award, which he was successful in obtaining. The award included about

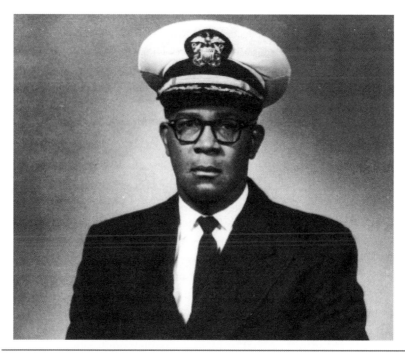

Commander Chester Pierce, U.S. Naval Reserve, circa 1965.

$10,000 that was allocated specifically to allow Chet to travel to other programs and familiarize himself with what other university centers were doing, both inside and outside their laboratories. So he seized the opportunity to visit colleagues at such places as Columbia University, McGill University, the University of Rochester, the University of Colorado, Tulane University, the University of Washington, UCLA, and the University of Oklahoma, and he even went to Mexico. He credits these trips with giving him substantial exposure to the field of psychiatry and influencing him to read the literature differently. It was also on these trips that he met academic luminaries such as Hans Selye, Heinz Lehmann, and Jolyon West, who was ultimately to play an important role in Chet's academic development during his Oklahoma years.

Chet wasted no time in making good use of the expertise that other faculty, who were well established in the department, could offer him. He liked the assignments that Maurice Levine gave him and which were clearly intended to deepen his all-around knowledge of psychiatry, particularly those that made use of his flair for general medicine. Don Ross was a helpful mentor who supervised his travel grant and made it easy for him to meet distinguished colleagues. Chet recalled with pleasure how Ross arranged for him to visit Mexico and even set it up so that Chet would give a lecture there. Chet saw it as a model for how contacts could really be helpful. Roy Whitman was a psychoanalyst who quickly became a collaborator. The two of them obtained a grant from the NIMH and set up a sleep laboratory. While Chet continued to explore questions that had to do with the general phenomenon of sleep, Whitman, as an analyst, was interested in waking people up so that he could deal more directly with their dreams.

Indeed, Chet's Cincinnati department was full of analysts, and they all trooped to Chicago for their training or as teachers. Chet felt the inexorable pressure to apply to an analytic institute, and with maximum ambivalence and hesitancy, he submitted the application form. A professor in the department had suggested to him that his entering treatment as a patient would facilitate smooth sailing of his application. Not surprisingly, Chet balked at that, no doubt seeing such an action as an infringement on his freedom and independence. Against his better judgment, he went off to Chicago for the required entrance interviews. One interviewer asked him to describe a favorite patient, and Chet responded by talking about a Black gangster's girlfriend he was treating. Chet thought he had probably stepped over the line by painting a picture of relative familiarity, by admitting that he liked the patient and enjoyed her jokes and general manner of interaction. When another interviewer asked Chet how old he was when his father abandoned the family, Chet, with that cold clenching of the jaw that I can detect only occasionally, explains to me that he just told him the truth about Samuel, who of course was devoted to his wife and sons all his life. The final question about whether he thought he should be in treatment was no doubt the straw that broke the camel's back. He gave his frank view of that and then returned home to await the rejection letter he knew was sure to come. Chet concluded that the interviewers were racist, and he also thought there was a tone to the exchanges that suggested that the interviewers were mulling over the question of whether Blacks could really be analyzed. I can readily imagine the analysts defending themselves by asserting that the major problem was Chet's and not theirs. I can also easily see them suggesting that Chet partly sabotaged the interviews, a claim that I think has some truth in it. Chet obviously had some inkling of the enormous sacrifice of time, energy, and money that analytic training required. But probably of greatest import to Chet was the fact that a group of White analysts would, through the analytic training process, have controlled his time, space, and energy, ultimately trying to impose their sense of discipline on him. So he was not disappointed when he received their rejection, and he started considering whether it was wise for a nonanalyst to contemplate a serious future at Cincinnati. Chet reports that, years later, Roy

Whitman told him that someone from the analytic institute had conceded that they made a mistake in rejecting Chet.

In my own generation of psychiatrist trainees, I have met several Blacks and other minorities who were enamored of the analytic tradition. But I knew instinctively I could never accept the rigid and sanctified discipline imposed on applicants to the analytic schools. I also knew that, regardless of the consequences, I could never bare my innermost thoughts to White men who were seated in explicit positions of authority and superiority with respect to me. And when in discussion one day with an analyst teacher who, in response to my question, replied confidently that I could not have enough money to buy a house in the select area in which he lived, I was instantly suspicious of analysis—as though a single swallow made an entire spring. But when later during an elective period at a distinguished New York hospital, a whole group of analysts conspired to make it clear to me I was merely a tolerated outsider at their hospital, I realized it would be especially difficult for me to become one of them. I also know it is patently silly to conclude that all analysts have difficulty in relating to Blacks, especially since some of my dearest colleagues have turned out to be analysts. But organized psychoanalysis has been arrogant in its response to the racial question, which has left me unforgiving in turn.

Of course, Cincinnati was also the place where Chet both deepened and broadened his other interests. He became fascinated by space, and he joined a national group of individuals who became formal observers of the Russian *Sputnik* as it passed overhead. He also developed a taste for community service and started serving on different committees. He recounts with fervor an experience with the National Conference for Christians and Jews. That group hosted a dinner each year and sold tables to benefit the organization. At a particular planning meeting, one man simply asked to be responsible for $15,000 worth of tables, but then went on to say that a colleague who was absent would also be guarantor for a substantial sum. Chet was dumbfounded. He didn't understand how one man could spend another's money, especially in his absence. Chet wondered whether that could happen among Blacks. Did Blacks have that kind of money, trust each other that much, and also feel that committed to any particular cause? Chet was also further struck by how little the group ever talked about Black people. Yes, tickets to the dinner were made available so that some members of the Black community could attend the dinner. But that did little to dampen Chet's concern that Blacks were really quite peripheral to the discussions of the group and had minimal impact on the group's policy decisions. What really frustrated Chet was his realization that these Whites didn't hate

Blacks; they just never thought about Black people. As a result, Blacks had no impact on the Whites' thinking.

This theme is important to Chet, and he doesn't let go of it easily. He connects it to an episode that occurred when he lived in Oklahoma. Senator Robert Kennedy, a college classmate and teammate, came through, visiting a rich family Chet knew. Like Chet, the family was also involved with Oklahoma's Kennedy Library Committee. The ostensible purpose of the group's meeting was to raise money for the library project, but it was hardly discussed at all. By the time the deadline rolled around, a member of the committee simply said he would donate the amount that they were expected to raise. Chet was surprised that so little effort was required to solve some of these fiscal problems. What seemed daunting to him turned out once again to be readily manageable in the eyes of others. The obvious implication, too, was that there were few Blacks, nationally, to be found in this league, and Chet realized how naive his perspective was on these types of issues.

As a general principle, Chet saw Cincinnati as a city that considered itself in the 1950s as the gateway to the South; as a result, relationships between the races were strained. Chet recalls that at the time there was a struggle over the opening of a public amusement park because before that time, parks had not been open to Blacks. Chet thinks that the Whites' emphasis on keeping Blacks away from the parks had lots to do with keeping Blacks out of the swimming pools located in the parks. That was, in turn, related to Whites' fear of being "contaminated" by the "dirt" that would necessarily be washed off the Blacks who went into the water. These Whites apparently feared the consequences of close contact with Blacks without much clothing.

Once he joined the faculty, Chet was involved in some of these community disputes, and his level of participation in civil rights activities increased when he moved to Oklahoma. He also points out that Patsy had a solid appreciation of all this. New Orleans, her hometown, was still segregated at that time, and she and Chet had shared the experience of traveling on segregated trains in the South. Chet also has never forgotten the trauma of going with Patsy to a movie theater located in a Cincinnati suburb, only to be greeted by a White woman who said, "I'd prefer that you not come in." It was in this context of becoming more aware of the participatory role in the Black-White struggle that Chet wrote his first paper on the subject of race relations while he was still in Cincinnati.

Chet's medical practice was, however, protected from discriminatory influences. He saw private patients at Christian Holmes Hospital, which was where all university doctors saw their private patients. Chet actually saw more White patients than Black ones, which bore testimony to the fact that his White colleagues were systematically referring patients to him.

Without wanting to dwell on it excessively, I still am curious about how Chet coped with these instances of mundane microtrauma, and I try to explore some more his reactions to such repeated discrimination. Chet makes it clear that such interactions with Whites were common at the time and that his responses varied. He describes a discussion with his daughter Diane, who was then learning to read. She was trying to decipher a sign she had seen when they stopped at a gas station in Alabama. So she asked Chet what the difference was between White ladies and colored women. He doesn't recall the answer he gave Diane, but he certainly remembers the feeling of being "demeaned, belittled, and emasculated." On the same trip, his car got stuck in a ditch off a country road in Alabama. He went to the closest house seeking help. A White man answered, and Chet explained his plight. The man then went across the road, knocked, and hollered at the Black occupant of the house to come on out and bring a chain. The Black man complied, and the two of them freed the car. Chet observed that the Black man never said a word; he just shuffled along quietly. Although Chet has never forgotten the paradox of generosity and cruelty in the same act, he made no comment about it at the time.

Chet's insightful observations on race lead him to tell me yet another story. He and Patsy were used to traveling on segregated trains where they had to go to the dining car to eat. They were served but had to take their meal behind a black curtain. Chet makes an association to the time he was taking a plane trip to the South Pole with an admiral aboard. He recalled that this high-ranking officer was separated from everyone else by a black curtain. Chet burst out laughing at the juxtaposition of these two vignettes that reductionistically ask what's behind a black curtain. He points out that human beings will go to considerable lengths to establish and maintain the concept of difference. He's flooded by one more memory, this time of his family taking a trip together and staying at the only hotel in the District of Columbia that would admit them. The incident has stuck in his mind because of the hotel's striking name, the Whitelaw Hotel.

Although he hasn't been able to efface the memories, time, humor, patience, and common sense have helped him to put them into perspective and to recognize that race in this country *does* matter. No wonder, then, that he and I repeatedly return to a cardinal theme in his political schema: that a Black can never truly belong to any predominantly White organization in this country. Chet is definitive in his declaration when he adds, "I believe that and I teach that. That's also what I was

taught by my father." Chet knows of my special interest in this phenomenon of belonging, and I know he senses my displeasure at his invoking
the regal presence of his father. It is hard enough to take on Chet in this
argument, but I say to myself that I cannot fairly be expected to fight
against a whole other generation too. At any rate, I throw his father's
image right back at him when I point out, with a modicum of taunting,
that Samuel's whole objective was to make sure that one day his sons
could join the Glen Cove country club and earnestly feel they belonged
there. Chet concedes that his father certainly wanted them to be able to
compete, but he concludes our argument that day with the declaration,
"I don't know what it would feel like to belong." As a sort of after-
thought, he explains that he was recently present at a reunion of his
Harvard football team and he got up and left before the end of the cer-
emonies. The feeling of not belonging was too powerful. The strength
of the sentiment makes it clear we'll see it again.

As I said, I am much taken by this notion of belonging, partly because it is a significant by-product of the interaction between dominant
and nondominant groups, a central theme in my preoccupation with
cultural psychiatry. In my mind I go back to the occasion when I was
conducting a workshop on ethnicity and intergroup relations at the
Houston campus of the University of Texas. I asked the group to react
to a passage I had read from Piri Thomas's autobiography that centered
on his asking a White high school student to dance. She not only refused
his invitation but then told a White friend that Black Piri had had nerve
in asking her to dance. In reaction to the passage, a Black member of the
audience spoke up and expressed amazement that Thomas had not
simply stayed with the Blacks at the dance. Instead, Thomas had gone
courting rejection, especially since, in this member's view, Black
women were much better dancers. At the time, I fought hard to control
my laughter, partly because I had not expected such brazen assertion of
group solidarity based on stereotype or myth. But this Black individual
in the audience was also giving voice to his conceptual view of life. He
recognized that he did not belong to the White group and he therefore
sought solace and friendship among his own. It is an important answer
to questions about the interplay of the dominant White and nondominant Black groups in the United States. Although I know I do not agree
with this stance, I still must recognize its power and force.

One particular year of Chet's faculty stay at the University of Cincinnati deserves special mention because it was then that chronic illness
became part of his family life. Chet is clear about protecting his family's
right to privacy, and I respectfully turn away my prying eyes and hold
my tongue. But my silence invites him to muse about his inability to

take on the pain of his loved ones so that they might suffer less. This time, in contrast to the almost imperceptible clenching of the jaw, I think I see a flicker of a tear in Chet's eyes, and I sense the deep sorrow this has caused him. I move on to yet another profoundly painful event, the death of Hettie in 1958.

Chet's mother died in a tuberculosis sanatorium on Long Island, where she had been hospitalized for about 2 or 3 years, suffering from that dreaded pulmonary disease as well as diabetes. Burton had called to tell Chet about their mother's deterioration, but Chet didn't see her before she died. She had first taken seriously ill when he was in the Navy. It turned out that Burton was the designated caregiver of Hettie in those final years, although neither Chet nor Burton could explain to me how the choice of caregiver actually occurred. In lots of families, it often turns out to be the last child; in others, it is the female who ends up with the task; and in still others, it is determined by geographic proximity. Later in the conversation, Chet thinks that may well have been the explanation because Burton was the only one at home in Glen Cove before Hettie went to the sanatorium.

At my unrelenting insistence, Chet offers the explanation that it was simply the luck of the draw, and he adds the almost gratuitous comment that Burton never asked for relief. But Chet must know I have questions about what I see as Hettie's obvious separation and her apparent isolation from her "baby boy" in her final years, and I am beside myself when he can recall no particular themes in any of their contacts once he married Patsy. Of course, sons and daughters are different, but still…. Hettie's funeral service took place at the Calvary AME Church in Glen Cove, and she was interred alongside her husband in Cold Spring Harbor. Chet sums it all up when he allows that he retains greater memory of his father's death a decade earlier than of his mother's passing in 1958. The three boys still get together once a year to place a flower on their parents' graves, a ritual that apparently got started as a result of a commitment given to their father before he died.

By 1960, Chet was 33 years old, a time when he would, in Levinsonian terms once again, have been completing the age-thirty transition and looking to settle down and construct a second adult life structure. His first adult life structure would have taken in the period of his early and middle twenties, when he was a "novice adult" and essentially involved in carrying out his basic and advanced medical studies. Levinson hypothesized that men in the age-thirty transition contemplate the flaws in their present life, with an eye to making corrections that lead to greater satisfaction, a more positive sense of being serious and settled, and connection to a niche they can justifiably call their own.

It was therefore understandable that Chet began to consider making a change, even though he felt he was doing very well at Cincinnati. I press the point and ask him to reflect on what catalyzed his thinking. Chet recounts a story that is quite revealing. One day a secretary in the Department of Psychiatry asked him whether he had received a memorandum of some sort that had been circulated, and he said that he hadn't. She thought that was strange because it had been sent to all the trainees. By that time, he had been on the faculty for several years. He felt "infantilized" and also concluded that the secretary's behavior was typical. He was convinced that faculty joining the department from outside training programs would be seen differently and that his advancement would be constrained because he would always be seen to be too "familiar." He would therefore consistently lack a certain status and dignity, even though he knew that the secretary was personally fond of him.

But there were other reasons to consider leaving Cincinnati. He was impatient to be more independent and to do what he wanted. For example, he experienced too many bureaucratic checks on him, too many layers to go through in setting up the courses he wanted to teach. The department had only four or five full professors, and he could see that advancement would be slow because the slots at the top were limited. Additionally, many job offers were coming to him. But we turn back to the issue of his rejection by the psychoanalytic institute, and he concedes that the rejection cast a cloud over his head in the department. In retrospect, he felt that the analysts constituted too much of a "religion." He permits himself an insightfully biting comment when he remarks that the analytic manner of talking about a specific Black patient in abject poverty and worrying about how her mother treated her was nonsense. Chet concedes he had "resistance" to some of the ideas the analysts were pushing, and he was also sure that his attitude toward analysis was evident to his supervisors and mentors. Still, when talking about his ultimate decision to leave and go to Oklahoma, he notes that "By fortune, I made a good selection." He remains persuaded that by leaving Cincinnati, his academic career moved ahead 10 years, even though he obviously could not have predicted that at the time.

Chet reminds me that a former Black colleague of ours named Charles Wilkinson, who died a few years ago, had been at a state hospital in Cincinnati in the 1950s and had left to go to Kansas City. Chet and he had become good friends, and Charlie had invited Chet to consider joining him in Missouri. Before he made up his mind, Chet received an invitation from Jolyon West, chairman of the Department of Psychiatry at the University of Oklahoma, to look at what Oklahoma had to offer. Professor West was, of course, someone whom Chet had met during his travels that were supported by the NIMH Career Teacher's Award, and Chet knew that West was himself interested in sleep physiology and in broader questions of consciousness. There was a natural and exciting fit, so the die was cast.

Chet and Patsy were soon on their way to Oklahoma even though she had not seen the university's campus. He understatedly says she just had faith in his decisions. But it prompts me to review with him the nature of his love and family relationships at the time of his age-thirty transition. By the time he left for Oklahoma, Diane was about 7 years old and Deirdre was about 2. He affirms that both he and Patsy were firmly into raising the two children and that child-rearing was definitely a part of their collective happiness. He retrospectively comments that for him, marriage and his children always came first, and when he was at home and not traveling, he always made an effort to be consciously attentive to them.

At such moments we both sit reflectively pondering our own thoughts. Chet goes on to muse about some of the contrasting cultural styles that characterize Black men and White men. We talk about Chet's being at a conference, sitting around chatting with some White male colleagues, when one chap pointedly boasts how some prostitutes had accosted him. He clearly made the assumption that one of the women had found him pleasing to her eye. Chet thinks the woman had identified the colleague as someone who would pay her price. In a clear spirit of unadulterated Black male chauvinism, we both agree that a Black brother would only have opened up his mouth to boast that the woman had offered herself free of charge. We burst out laughing, as much at our outrageous claims as at our professed sociological insights.

Wishing to summarize other issues that relate to the age-thirty transition, I ask Chet about the notions of forming a dream and developing mentor relationships, techniques that often serve to help us deconstruct the longitudinal development of a particular individual. Chet is unable to see any dream take form. He thinks his movement and choices were haphazard. He was never sure of where he was going, although he believed in living fully. Even the goal of being a Black psychiatrist was at the time murky in his mind, and in 1960 it wasn't even evident that Blacks could actually make a living at that kind of work. Acknowledging that "we're all hostages to our times," Chet thinks he just wanted to be in the right place at the right time, which by definition would put him in an "upward draft." So he would be constantly advancing and going upward. Added to that, the most exciting things in his life came unexpectedly. It is in this positive frame of mind that he opted to make the move to Oklahoma, to settle down and build the new life structure.

Chet agrees with the idea that it is important to have senior people in your life who will teach you, advocate on your behalf, and even protect you at important points along the way. We review the names of individuals already mentioned who had been an important part of his success in the Navy. We turn then to Cincinnati, and he repeats the names of Roy Whitman and Donald Ross, while adding the names of Charles Hofling and Louis Gottschalk, who taught him about verbal analysis and patient care. Chet can't help lamenting his concern that it may be easier for Whites to find and connect to important mentors than it is for aspiring young Black students.

In my case, the change in my age-thirty transition came as I decided in 1977 to leave New York and join the Yale faculty in New Haven. In retrospect, I clearly had the dream of becoming a university professor, although I was not yet sure what my particular interest in psychiatry would be. But I agree with Chet about the distinct influence of chance on the decisions made. My choice of Yale was a clear function of my wife's already being there, although her decision had been forced by other circumstances beyond her control. There is also no question that mentors have played well-defined roles at every phase of my adult career.

4

The Oklahoma Years

In 1960, Chet and Patsy drove to Oklahoma with their older daughter, Diane, and left Deirdre with Patsy's parents for about a month so that the settling-in period could proceed without the additional difficulty of their having to care for a very young child. After a week in a segregated motel, they rented a house close to the medical school. Chet reminds me again that those were "segregated times" and no other option existed. In Oklahoma City, Blacks not only couldn't eat downtown in certain restaurants, they also couldn't try on clothes in most stores. When I raise the question, Chet can't remember whether he and Jolyon West discussed these social conditions when he was being recruited for the position. However, he does remember that in his first week at work, West and he successfully tested a public pool that had never before welcomed a Black swimmer. Being prevented by law from living or eating somewhere is an aspect of life I have never experienced as an adult, and I wonder how I would react to the necessity of accepting such conditions. I expect that where no real option exists, one can learn to swallow more bitter pills than racial segregation, which in a certain sense may not be the worst of extreme environments after all.

Chet started his new job as assistant professor of psychiatry and assistant chief of the Department of Psychiatry at the Oklahoma Veterans Administration Hospital. He was full of enthusiasm, and he recalls vividly not only the vibrancy of the staff but the solid research orientation of the department. The staff included Jolyon West, who had a major interest in sleep research and in brainwashing; Jay Shurley, a psychoana-lyst and specialist in sensory deprivation; Eugene Pumpian-Mindlian, vice-chairman of the department and a master clinician; Boyd Lester, a sleep researcher; Hal Williams, a research psychologist; Robert Edel-berg, a psychophysiologist; Oscar Parsons, who was interested in brain changes caused by flickering lights; and Vladimir Pishkin, a research psychologist. To these names, Chet adds two more individuals: James Mathis, a former general practitioner who became Chet's research col-laborator; and Jim Stuart, a friend from the Navy who had joined the Oklahoma faculty. In recalling names, Chet mentions George Lythcott, the Black pediatrician and part-time faculty member whom Chet had known since Chet's own adolescent years. Lythcott was a strong source of support for Chet in those early years and later went on to become a medical school dean in New York City.

By 1962, Jay Shurley had vacated the leadership of psychiatry at the VA Hospital and taken a research professorial position in the depart-ment. Consequently, with the support of Shurley and West, Chet was promoted to fill Shurley's old spot and was also made director of resi-dency training for the department. He lectured to first-year medical stu-dents on the behavioral sciences and also started a day center for certain psychiatric patients. He proceeded, too, to unlock his inpatient services and to encourage employees from all over the hospital to come visit the psychiatric wards so that they would have a better sense of what mental illness was all about. Opening the wards took a lot of effort, and Chet recalls that he did it on his mother's birthday, April 5, 1962.

Still a member of the Navy Reserve, Chet maintained connections to the Navy's psychiatric research unit in San Diego. At the time, the re-searchers were working on how individuals adapt to prisoner-of-war status and to other peculiarly stressful contexts, such as being stationed in Antarctica. Knowing of Chet's continuing interest in sleep, they sug-gested that Chet ought to visit Antarctica, and he promptly began to discuss the idea with Jay Shurley. The Antarctic offered itself as a natu-ral laboratory for studying questions of geology, physics, and climatol-ogy; it also tested the capacity of humans to adapt to stress. The interests of Chet and Jay Shurley could easily coalesce in an Antarctic project because Shurley was studying stress and deprivation, and Chet's work on sleep was relevant to the hypothesis that humans living in the Antarctic region spent less time sleeping than did humans else-where. So Chet made an exploratory visit to the region in 1963, and on his return to the university, he and Shurley spent a year developing plans for their joint research project that would focus on how humans adjust to the extreme, isolated, confined conditions of the South Pole.

Their idea was first to study a group of volunteers who would be housed at a base in Rhode Island and therefore living at sea level. These same individuals would be followed for a year while serving at the South Pole and for 6 months after their return to the United States. These differing living conditions would enable some comparison to be made of the study group's sleep patterns and to clarify whether the changes in sleep were accompanied by any compromise in the individuals' functioning. The researchers were also interested in what particular psychological elements had impact on the adaptation of the group to their spartan living conditions and in the responses of the body to the changed physical environment. This study would be done by examining the group members' quality and quantity of sleep, their dreams, and biological studies of different blood and urine parameters.

They presented their ideas to the National Science Foundation and received funding for their study, with Shurley as the principal investigator and Chet as co-principal investigator on the project. Their plan was to set up a laboratory at the geographic South Pole right in the middle of the Antarctic; they did not intend that they themselves should stay there for any extended period of time. It was not necessary for them to stay there because they had no lack of volunteers from among the medical students to help carry out the studies, which were ultimately published after Chet moved to Harvard in 1968.

Chet thinks it important at this point to delineate in some detail the feasibility visit that he made to the South Pole in 1963 for a 3-month period. He immediately mentions the strong support provided by Jolyon West, who asked only that his department be acknowledged when the study results were published. Chet agrees that times were different then and that the academic culture allowed him to be absent from work for such an extended period. In fact, Chet points out that even on the trip down he wasn't sure of the return date because it would depend on the weather.

He recalls that he left the States the same day President John Kennedy was assassinated. He traveled as a civilian for the National Science Foundation, and the Air Force flew him from the District of Columbia to Honolulu, then to New Zealand, and from there to McMurdo Base in the Antarctic, the first landing site. The Americans had bases located elsewhere, along with those of other countries. But only the United States was at the South Pole, where Chet spent most of his time on this first visit, in the company of about 30 men who lived 40 feet under the ice. At that time, no women were there. Chet visited Byrd Station, Plateau Station, the Dry Valleys, and a New Zealand base, and he worked at a penguin rookery. He recalls tagging penguins so that their movements could be monitored over time; also, seals were being studied to see whether they were a possible reservoir of psittacosis. The tenor of some of the discussions with his colleagues there didn't fail to strike Chet as odd, such as the occasion when they spent an hour discussing whether they ought to block out the light so that they could sleep. But Chet thinks that knowing he would eventually leave helped him cope with the harshness of the environment and the phenomenon called density clustering, which had to do with the effects produced on people by their forced interaction with others under extreme environmental conditions.

Keeping himself balanced allowed Chet to focus more clearly on the purpose of his visit, which was to find a site where they could set up the laboratory. Chet found that mundane issues suddenly became important, such as where could one ground an EEG machine when ground was 9,000 feet away and covered by ice, or where could someone wash his hands easily. Indeed, the lack of running water meant that someone always had to be awake and alert to the possibility of fires. Chet exercised rigorously, then went to a room filled with steam flowing from odd pipe fittings. He also spent time listening to all sorts of music and reading voraciously.

Chet remarks, without elaborating much more about it, that Patsy had observed a difference in his behavior before he left. This is apparently a commonly observed phenomenon among those contemplating a stressful venture, such as a trip to an extreme environment, although it has been little studied. He adds, too, that Patsy did support his making the trip, which is in itself an interesting sidelight of the experience. Chet points out that in work he did later in the Arctic among participants in a long-distance dogsled race, he found that competitors who lacked the enthusiastic support of their mates did not finish in the top half of the group. So he believed Patsy's endorsement was important. I smile at the familiar reality that so many of us are successful in our achievements only because there is the solid support of a partner facilitating our quest to channel our energies in a specific direction.

Chet explains that he ultimately decided the South Pole base was the best location for the work. The investigators needed instrumentation that would contribute to the strong science basis of the research; indeed, whatever they did needed to be scientific in order for them to gain the trust and cooperation of the other researchers at the South Pole. In addition, the human volunteers had to be monitored carefully so as to minimize their tendency to sabotage a research study conducted in that sort of environment.

In his associative style, Chet goes on to talk about something that occurred after a 1966 trip to the South Pole, where he had let his beard grow. He was sitting in the Dallas airport, waiting to change planes,

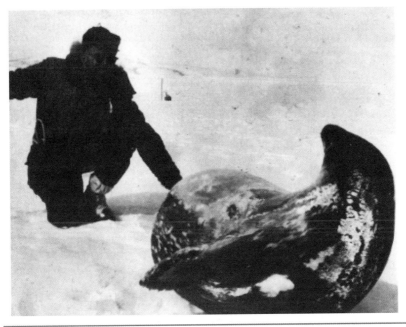

Chester Pierce approaches a seal in Antarctica, 1963.

when a stranger walked up to him and started berating him, obviously taking Chet for some sort of antiwar beatnik or hippie. The man was White and clearly upset by Chet's beard and by the fact that the man's son was in Vietnam while Chet was still in the States. Chet's response was instantaneous anger. It is unusual to hear Chet talk about being angry—ever—but then he goes on to explain how he actually pondered the thought of hurting the stranger if the stranger had touched him! Jay Shurley, who had missed much of the exchange, appeared on the scene and explained to the stranger that in fact Chet was a military veteran who had already served in the armed forces. The stranger then sheepishly apologized and went on his way. Chet points out that he has been that angry only two or three times in his whole life, and he clearly recalls his registering the thought that he was certainly back in the United States. The episode highlights the crucial impact of the race matter on the psychological terrain of Chet Pierce and the potential explosiveness of the cumulative experience of discrimination. No doubt, his patience and usual emotional control were also worn a bit thin during the extended time he had just spent in the extreme environment. But the confrontation reveals a special vulnerability that belies the steady calm that so characterizes the man and exposes a seething anger that makes him seem all the more human. Something about the racist politics of the

United States can actually get under his skin, and with frightening intensity. Chet concedes that the episode troubled him because it reminded him of his own vulnerability, which for the most part he controls and hides well.

But I sense that in addition to the understandable fear of his potential explosiveness, there is something problematic about having his deepest emotions called forth by a White male who had little real connection to Chet's everyday life. The context also was relatively trivial, since the Vietnam war issue was not central to anything Chet was involved with at the time. Of course, seen from another vantage point, these were all reasons the unknown White male's entrance into Chet's private space was perceived by Chet as such a hostile act. The man lacked any standing, so to speak, that justified his deliberate intrusiveness, unless one grasps Chet's likely view that Whites often claim standing to intervene by virtue of their asserted superiority over Blacks. The random, apparently haphazard interaction of that White man and Chet can therefore be recast into a predictable experience that was logically and arrogantly set up by the racialist culture of the United States.

It is an event such as that one that explicates Chet's notion of racism as an environmental pollutant, as a problem with broad public health consequences. All the actors in the drama have been stained by the polluting effects of the racialist culture. In this specific instance, the White perpetrator of the metaphorical assault can go forward with his action because his racial superiority justifies it. Chet responds angrily because he sees the White man's act as more than a father's anger at the injustice of war and an unfair draft system. Chet's own thinking is polluted by the impact of racism. The remaining problem, of course, is how to decontaminate everybody, a question with substantive futuristic implications.

It is misleading, however, to frame Chet Pierce's experiences with racism or rejection solely as part of the context of the United States. He takes me back to a 1963 trip to New Zealand, a country he had passed through several times and that had welcomed him graciously in the past. On this particular visit, he returned to his hotel room from shopping and found a card identifying him as Unwanted Alien #39 and instructing him to carry the card at all times. Chet naturally wondered whether some administrative error had been made, but he was in no mood to find out. He angrily called the National Science Foundation representative in New Zealand, raised hell about his treatment, and then demanded to be put on the next flight out of the country. The representative advised him to go to the airline office to obtain the ticket. Chet did just that, found the ticket all ready for him, and received help from an airline official who, from shame and embarrassment, invited

Chet to dinner that night. In no mood to be mollified, Chet turned down the invitation, left the airline office with his ticket in hand, and promptly got lost. The story would be any psychoanalyst's delight. In the midst of his anger and confusion, Chet ran into a Black American engineer from Kansas who was married to a British woman and owned a nightclub in New Zealand. The man took Chet to dinner and introduced Chet to his wife. A friendship developed, and Chet became godfather to their next child. Chet ultimately learned what a difficult time the American had had building a life in New Zealand. For example, when he had first expressed an interest in marrying a White woman, he ended up in a mental hospital! Chet found out later that even some of his New Zealand friends were not aware the country had an unwanted alien policy that served to keep the country White.

I wasn't surprised by his vignette because I recalled how difficult it was for me to obtain a student visa to study at an Australian medical school in the summer of 1971. With all my expenses guaranteed, including my departure from the country to return to my medical studies, the Australians weren't pleased that I was born in the Caribbean and was obviously Black. It was my first encounter with bureaucratic, governmental racism, and I have never forgotten it. Amusingly enough, when I was finally let into the country after an aggressive intervention from friends, the average Australian was extremely gracious and hospitable. The stay turned out to be among my most pleasant international trips. But I pondered long and hard the feeling of being classified as an unwanted person because I was Black. The whole thing kept its own private meaning for me years later when I heard Chet, in a lecture at Yale, insist he has never been to any country in the West where there wasn't significant categorization based on race or color. He followed it up with the thought that he has never lived an adult day without having to think about race matters. I recall the lecture well and can still hear the stunning silence. Australia came crashing back to me because it characterized the international nature of the problem, once again clearly highlighted for me in the early 1980s on a trip to Colombia as a Kellogg Foundation National Fellow. My hosts took me to visit farms, health clinics, and educational institutions. It was clear that Colombians came in all hues. But then we went to a dinner for the elite, and suddenly Colombia was all White. I didn't think it mattered until a Colombian friend told me there was no color distinction in the country. I decided he was either blind or puerile, and I moved on. Chet and I leave this topic for the time being and return to the discussion about Oklahoma.

Jay Shurley, Jolyon West, and Chet collaborated in their work on the general phenomenon of consciousness as seen in their individual thinking about sleep, sensory deprivation, and brainwashing. Shurley's work actually shed light on how people react differently in the stressful context of an environment bereft of usual sensory stimulation such as sound and light. The specific model used was the placement of a volunteer under water in a darkened tank. Chet himself responded quite well to the experience but readily contrasted it with the bizarre reactions he observed in others. He had also tested female pilots in the tank, candidates for the astronaut program. They performed impressively, as Chet very well expected them to do. But he also recalls his hunch at the time that the female applicants were only being put through the testing motions and would not finally be accepted for astronaut training, and he was right.

I am curious about what Chet thinks were primary factors in assuring the stability of an individual experiencing sensory deprivation in the tank. He responds that prior knowledge of what would happen and the capacity to structure thinking were two important characteristics. Structured thinking refers to staying systematically occupied and busy with one's own thoughts. So, for example, someone in the tank could simply ignore the conditions of being immersed in water in the dark and could then concentrate on developing a budget in his head for the coming year. The sensory deprivation work served me well years later when I was studying a new religious group in the Caribbean that used sensory deprivation techniques in a Christian ritual. The particular ceremony consisted of having group members be isolated for a week in a section of the church with their eyes banded to keep out light and cotton wool in their ears to exclude sound. After the ritual was over, participants would report to the larger congregation gathered at a special Sunday service that they had experienced special visions and had traveled to strange lands and seen Jesus and other prophets. Those who recounted very graphic images generally had some prior knowledge about the ritual. But clearly, the individual capacity to structure one's thinking facilitated a process of relaxation that in turn catalyzed the focusing on religious themes that the group traditionally prized so highly.

Some of Chet's work on sleep that he had carried out in Cincinnati began to see print in the early sixties. This work had been influenced by other researchers working on eye movements that occurred during sleep, who had hypothesized that the eye movements were associated with dreaming. Chet therefore wondered whether individuals with enuresis dreamed about water at the time they actually wet the bed and also whether they were in a period of light or heavy sleep at the time they urinated. These questions were particularly intriguing because many people with the disorder had reported that they wet the bed while dreaming of urinating. Therefore, because they were thought to have some form of sleep pathology, the question was whether one could clarify the nature of the pathology by understanding better the quality and frequency of their dreams.

Chet and his colleagues described the results of 20 nights when their research subjects wet the bed while in the laboratory. On those occasions, bedwetting and dreaming never occurred together. Generally, the initial dream occurred after the first episode of bedwetting, and the EEG tracings confirmed that in the majority of cases the subjects were in deep sleep when they wet the bed. Such results led Chet to the theory that bedwetting was usefully conceptualized as a form of sleep disorder, that the dream mechanism in individuals with the disorder was likely out of phase, and that enuresis was a dream substitute or dream equivalent. Consequently, it was a natural next step to seek more biological and psychological data about those with the disorder. It seemed reasonable to look for biological correlates, such as cholesterol levels taken throughout the night from those with the disorder, and to study the relationship of children with the disorder to their mothers.

It was in Oklahoma that Chet looked to other clinical phenomena to provide more information about sleep. Such examples included bruxism, narcolepsy, and hydranencephaly. The hydranencephalic infant essentially has no brain, and the cranial cavity is occupied by cerebrospinal fluid. Chet's interest was in knowing whether someone without a brain could dream. Because he could not in reality expect the hydranencephalic infant to respond to the question, he was looking for the answer through a proxy method, which in this case was the EEG sleep levels and associated rapid eye movements when the individual was lightly asleep. A bit to his surprise, the results did show that rapid eye movements occurred in hydranencephaly. On the other hand, because these individuals were also blind and deaf, Chet theorized that it was doubtful the rapid eye movements were linked to the infants' experiencing formed images in a way that corresponded to what we usually mean in referring to the common phenomenon of dreaming. He also hypothesized that the basis of dreaming might be located in the brainstem.

It was at Oklahoma that Chet came to think of himself as the senior clinician/leader of a major psychiatric service. He had responsibility for a 75-bed unit, a day center, an outpatient service, and a service of consultation to other hospital wards. So Chet found himself trying to answer questions that arose in the context of his everyday administrative activity, and he often articulated his reflections in journal articles coauthored with different collaborators. He addressed the occupational therapy shop as a culture and argued that its improvement would hinge on bringing about changes in the occupational therapist–physician relationship. He examined barriers to research among pastoral counselors, and he looked at ways to attract general practitioners to clearer uses of psychiatric principles in their daily practices. Additionally, he wrote about music therapy.

Chet had actually addressed earlier the question of how one instilled career commitment in nursing personnel, recognizing that developing such commitment was as important as the initial recruitment of students into the profession of nursing. Chet and his nursing colleagues were evidently intrigued by the problem of nurse-physician relationships. They created the experimental situation in which a doctor directs a nurse to carry out a procedure that in some way runs contrary to the nurse's professional standards. By telephone, a ward nurse was asked by a doctor she did not know to give 20 mg of an oral medication to a patient, even though the maximum daily dosage was clearly marked on the box to be only 10 mg. Strict precautions were of course taken to ensure that the medication on the ward was in reality nothing but a placebo and that in fact the order was never carried out.

As it turned out, 21 of 22 nurses on the wards would have given the medication. In contrast, when the same scenario was presented in writing as a theoretical problem to a group of graduate nurses and a group of nursing students, the vast majority of them concluded that the medication should not be given. They cited appropriate reasons such as the fact that the medication dosage was excessive; they did not know the doctor; and there was no written order for the medication, which was clearly not being given in an urgent situation. The experimental context was intriguing for a number of reasons. It allowed a rare interdisciplinary and collaborative examination of problems in the nurse-physician relationship; in addition, the results of this experiment also must have been useful to Chet when he took over the major clinical services at Oklahoma. What he learned must certainly have facilitated his creating mutual trust on his clinical services and talking openly about factors that would have made it possible for so many nurses in practice to ignore important tenets of their profession and mistakenly accede to the physician's orders.

Chet progressively cultivated an interest in working with police officers, which was somewhat akin to the earlier work he had done with guards at the naval brig. He recalls that his chief psychologist, Vernon Sisney, was very popular in Oklahoma City and had been a police officer while he was completing his graduate work. So Chet's connections to the police gradually developed, supported by Jolyon West's idea that it was good for their department to have established linkages to the community. Indeed, it was West's idea that support groups be run for spouses of police officers. Chet enjoyed the special relationship he had with the chief of police, and he liked the long talks they engaged in. These chats were facilitated by Captain Gene Goold, who ultimately became one of Chet's best friends. The experience gave Chet the chance to reflect on different facets of the interaction between the police and Blacks and to appreciate the complexity of the policy road the chief had to walk. It is with at least a modicum of sympathy, then, that Chet explains the discussion with the chief about the wisdom of placing a Black police officer in downtown Oklahoma City. Both of them recognized that such a decision might well have resulted in the officer's having to direct White drivers, assist White ladies, and perhaps even arrest some White individual in full view of many other Whites—all of which would have doubtless been seen as deliberate provocation from the chief and additionally reflecting a lack of administrative judgment.

I feel a twinge of sympathy for the chief, and then Chet adds another dimension to the story about his discussions with the police chief. One day Chet and the chief were talking about the experiences of one of his patrolmen. A fracas had occurred, and the officer went to investigate. He approached a Black man sitting on the porch, relaxing with his legs up. For no reason, the officer struck the man's feet with the baton, and the man immediately jumped up, hopping on one foot. Not surprisingly, of course, the officer was at the wrong house, and it was an innocent man who received the blow. But the chief was laughing as he recounted this tale to Chet, and he didn't quite grasp the possible implications for Chet himself as a Black man, although the chief had displayed considerable sophistication in explicating the difficulties in stationing a Black police officer downtown. But here again was the phenomenon of environmental pollution. The chief had not even grasped the extent of the racism in the jocular narrative, nor had he appreciated the danger to his officers and the whole community that was reflected in the policeman's behavior.

Chet's relationship with Jolyon West was obviously an important source of both intellectual and psychological support, and Chet takes a certain pride and pleasure in describing his work with West on the famous elephant, the results of which were published in the prestigious journal *Science*. The story is unique because it at once captures the thinking of the two men while still showing that it was possible for Black and White to share space and time, even in light of the nature of Black-White relationships in the United States in the 1960s.

At the time, West was theorizing a lot about the unique environment and experience of being in captivity, and he planned to stage a departmental symposium on the subject. In keeping with the broad style of his thinking, West invited to the event several individuals he considered to be experts on captivity. They were the director of a local state hospital, a zoo director, and a senior police official. After the speeches, they were all chatting in West's office, and Chet engaged the zoo director in a discussion of the management of elephants in captivity. It is at first hard to follow the connectedness in the discourse, until Chet explains that they had all been interested in the lives of big animals, not only humans. Chet had also been consistently intrigued by historical events, and he knew that the Romans in ancient times were able to manage male elephants in captivity, but that in modern times there were in fact relatively few captive male elephants to be found, for example, in zoos. This was the result of the musth phenomenon, a period during which male elephants went wild, while discharging a sticky glandular substance. Jolyon West wanted to know what was in the substance and whether the substance might be excreted by an elephant that was in a state of chemical psychosis induced, for example, by the injection of LSD. The researchers were conceptualizing a fascinating experimental animal model. They wondered whether secretion of the substance was in fact synonymous with elephant psychosis, which was another way of saying that the elephant's deranged state was mediated through this endogenously secreted substance whose pharmacological makeup scientists ignored. I ask Chet whether the musth phenomenon had anything to do with the elephant's being in captivity, which is my way of trying to clarify the connection between the conference on captivity and the ensuing discussion about elephant behavior. There is no connection. The talk about the elephants simply came from a common interest in the management of big animals.

The zoo director, Dr. Warren Thomas, who later became director of the Los Angeles Zoo, arranged to have a male elephant transferred to the Oklahoma City Zoo, and the researchers developed a protocol for the experiment. At the same time, both because they had no idea of what dose of LSD to give the elephant and also because West was then studying psychedelics, they all took LSD themselves. Chet recalls that when he took the substance, he became "super polite," then went home and went to sleep. He woke up with startling clarity about a number of things, including the idea that a faculty member's wife had been impregnated at age 17 by a Black man. I laugh quietly and stifle the impulse to ask whether Chet was himself the obviously precocious young man, remembering that neither Hettie nor Samuel would likely have considered such a thought to be amusing.

After calculating what they thought was an appropriate dose, the researchers shot the elephant with LSD, and to their surprise, the animal began wobbling, fell down and broke off its tusk, then started showing signs of a seizure, accompanied by harsh, noisy breathing. They tried to revive the elephant using massive doses of Nembutal, in addition to other heroic measures, but to no avail. The elephant died, without producing enough of the substance for the researchers to study, although they were able to publish the changes in cell structure in relevant journals.

Chet could still enumerate a number of the lessons he had learned from the experience: about elephants and their care, particularly noting that they live as long as people do; about the behavior of large animals held in captivity; about what Chet calls speciesism—the lack of regard that humans have for other animals, which in turn partly accounts for the ease with which we treat other humans badly; about the notion that elephants receive much more basic care from their biological mother and from herd surrogates than humans receive, which raises fundamental questions about the longitudinal outcome for humans. Still, the researchers did not answer the questions about the relationship of the musth phenomenon to psychosis and captivity. Neither did they shed light on the role that sleep deprivation played in facilitating the onset of the maddened state. Animal psychosis was another subtext to the elephant story and one that was of particular interest to Chet.

While living in Oklahoma City, Chet became very interested in sit-ins, the well-known tool that Blacks were using at the time to advance their cause in the civil rights struggle. Before hastening to participate, Chet informed Jolyon West of his intentions, so as not to embarrass either West personally or the university. In fact, Chet points out with the utmost respect and affection that instead of letting him go alone to the demonstration, West accompanied him and clearly indicated support of Chet on this important political issue. At the 1964 Annual Meeting of the American Psychiatric Association, they presented a joint paper on the psychodynamic causes and effects of sit-ins and later published the paper. Of particular note was their finding that among the 300 regular sit-in demonstrators, who were usually adolescents or children, there were "no manifestations of delinquency or anti-social behavior, no school drop-outs, and no known illegitimate pregnancies…a remarkable record for any group of teenage children of any colour in any community in 1964." Chet and West realized that the demonstrators learned to appreciate the power they wielded over their White opponents and came to derive certain psychological benefits from their ordeals. In all fairness, Chet understood too that there were others participating in the sit-ins, such as "the starry-eyed idealists, the cynics, the professionals, the publicity-seekers, the sexual adventurers." Pierce, West, and Mathis became major participants in and advisers about sit-ins.

Talk of sit-ins reminds Chet of the time that Charlton Heston, who since the 1950s was the best friend of Jolyon West, visited Oklahoma City. The incident occurred around 1962 or 1963, while Heston was president of the Screen Actors Guild. Before Heston arrived, West announced that three men of "the same size and intelligence" were going to take a walk with sandwich boards protesting racism. West, Heston, and Chet did it, up and down Oklahoma City's Main Street, garnering enormous publicity. Chet still laughs at the whole scene and mockingly comments that it was little surprise, then, that the Psychiatry Department got the reputation of being more interested in race riots and elephants than in teaching psychiatry.

But Chet's admiration of the young people who participated in the civil rights work was genuine, and he has consistently felt the responsibility for giving thought to the welfare of each younger generation of Blacks. He speaks, therefore, with considerable pride about what he calls his Oklahoma People Program, which he set up with financial help from General Electric. The idea was to expose Black high school students to other Blacks younger than age 35 who were successful in unconventional occupations. Chet invited the founder of a computer firm, an astrophysicist, a female journalist from *Ebony*, a television news commentator, and an entertainment lawyer. These people talked to the students about their work to give the youngsters a broader view of what Blacks could hope to do with their lives and what was realistically possible for minorities in the United States. This is an issue that Chet and I discuss from time to time: the narrowness of vision that so many Black youth seem to have in conceptualizing their long-term potential. As serious sports enthusiasts, he in football and basketball and I in soccer, we both know well the futility of the dream that sports is the success ticket for Black youth.

During the time at Oklahoma, Chet continued his interest in sports-related thinking and was also appointed to the editorial board of *The Physician and Sportsmedicine*. There was widespread love of football at the university, and people wanted to know his opinions on certain coaching policies. He received numerous invitations to speak on sports-related matters, and his popularity in this domain seemed to grow, with the steady support of a major figure in the field at the time. That was Harvard's Dr. Thomas Quigley, who was one of the few surgeons in the country with a major interest in sports surgery and who had been team doctor for the football squad Chet had played on. A need for confidentiality and secrecy also led him to receive a number of referrals of athlete-patients from Oklahoma State University, another athletic powerhouse in the state. Soon, Chet was consulting to the National Football League. He recalls a speech he gave to the NFL at the time, raising in typical Pierce fashion the futuristic dilemma of their having to confront the increased use of drugs by professional athletes. As clinician and consultant, Chet went on to work with major league athletes from various sports, as well as elite individual athletes such as those participating in the Olympic Games.

It is clear that Chet had multiple and varied intellectual interests that he pursued with substantial passion. (One such interest was in the domain of programmed instruction that he pursued with his colleagues Mathis and Pishkin. They demonstrated that after 12 hours of programmed study, college seminarians were able to pass the psychiatry section of the National Medical Board Examination.) Chet had an insatiable curiosity about lots of things, and he followed leads and opportunities that presented themselves along the way, without attending much to the notion that any particular idea might very well be a distraction from some more central theme. Chet recognizes, without much prodding, that his way of conceptualizing scholarly work both at Cincinnati and at Oklahoma may not necessarily be a helpful model for current-day young academics. He contrasts his own career style with that of Jim Maas, a colleague at Cincinnati. Maas focused on specific and narrow questions of biology and pursued answers with a rigorous attention to detail, not allowing himself to deviate from rigidly defined objectives. However, Chet thinks that each man's personality and work must fit together if there is to be a concordance of productivity and happiness. Of course, the result was that Chet had his fingers in a multiplicity of pies, and he was broadly informed about many things. He is not sure that by today's standards he would be considered an expert in the areas about which he wrote.

So we turn then to one other domain of work that occupied Chet during his stay at Oklahoma. The Tarahumara Indians lived in Chihuahua, Mexico, and were the subject of an extensive anthropological study conducted by researchers from the University of Oklahoma. The inquiry was under the aegis of Clyde Snow, later to become a world authority on exhumations of persons killed in civil wars. Chet was intrigued by the Indians' lifestyle because they engaged in relatively little crime, and they ran 250-mile footraces that lasted several days. After the races, the group had a party called a *tesquinada*, at which they drank a beer called *tesquina* while socializing and engaging in networking and economic exchange. The footrace traversed a 25-mile circuit (10 laps) and lasted throughout the night. Chet saw it as an Indigenous example of a group's adaptation to a prolonged stressful exercise, and he was struck by how well they coped, particularly given the high altitude at which they ran.

Chet also came to understand that the group relied on a number of organizational techniques that made for the collective success of the enterprise. He noted that Tarahumara children could wander around without fear of being hurt or abused by strangers. In fact, other families would take them in and care for them without complaint. The Indians also used shamanistic rituals to cope with the advent of stress and anxiety. Chet explains how one of the runners, who was having some trouble, was referred to him by a shaman for care. It turned out that the athlete felt his diminished performance resulted from his having been bewitched. Chet smiles in telling how he used some ordinary face powder to rub on the man, who returned later to express his appreciation for Chet's effective intervention. However, Chet acknowledges he never knew if the patient was truly helped or was merely exceedingly gracious. Chet's work with the Tarahumara Indians reflects his sociological eye, as he made other observations about their isolation from modern technology as well as their success in resisting some of the corruption of modern-day America.

His eye for sociological detail most clearly emerges in his description of Bumpy Johnson, a famous Black racketeer of the period. Chet was having dinner with his brother Burton at a restaurant in Harlem in 1963. At the end of the meal, the waiter told them that Bumpy had paid their bill; Bumpy had done so as a gesture of appreciation for some favor a member of the Pierce family had done him. Over the years, Chet and Bumpy had many long talks together whenever Chet visited New York for some meeting or other. They were obviously drawn together as polar opposites, and Bumpy had decided to give Chet an education that could not be acquired in the professor's books. Bumpy's frame of reference was clearly different from Chet's, and Chet began to have a deeper appreciation of the true complexity of human beings and the occasional difficulty of distinguishing between good and bad. Chet also was seeing for the first time what could induce individuals to perform corrupt acts. While he reflects on this, Chet is prompted to exclaim that life is really not simple at all.

The contradictions inherent in his observations of Bumpy's thinking and acting were instructive, as was his realization of his own profound ignorance of what went on in the world around him. He saw Bumpy lend someone $18,000 in cash, heard Bumpy explain how important White males employed upper-class prostitutes on cruises, and attended carefully to Bumpy's explication of how many people "had a piece of the action" when a new restaurant opened. Also, Bumpy maintained a legitimate business in soaps and detergents. Chet was struck by his own feeling that as Bumpy talked there was still an additional hidden structure that contributed to the smooth organization of all the activity. So Chet understood that in some ways his lessons remained incomplete, but he made his decision to stay distant from it all.

Indeed, when Bumpy died of heart disease, he was about to open a string of fancy restaurants; at this juncture, Bumpy had made Chet an offer to participate in a deal related to this new project, knowing full well that Chet couldn't accept it. Their friendship lasted about 5 years and ended with Chet's attendance at Bumpy's funeral. Chet thinks at least one major thing Bumpy taught him was the profound uncertainty of knowing and defining the true reference points by which people live. Chet adds that the film *Hoodlum*, released in the summer of 1997, is about the lives of Bumpy Johnson and other racketeers of that era.

I wonder about Chet's fascination with the character of Bumpy, and I understand that Bumpy is the embodiment of another arena of Black life with which so few Black intellectuals really have any familiarity. Bumpy also represents the Black man who has made use of his profound insights about Whites and who understands the strengths and the weaknesses of White people. Bumpy is, of course, also an economic success, and in his own way he is but another Samuel Pierce Sr., using knowledge to manipulate a system so clearly dominated by Whites. Samuel understood that Whites would not as a general rule freely invite Blacks to the table of economic opportunity, and he found ways to push his way ever so gently to that table. There was art in executing the task of getting to the economic trough, as both Samuel and Bumpy knew that drawing attention to one's Black presence there could produce the unfortunate backlash of having the crowd coalesce in sealing off the Black intruder and blocking access. In one way, Bumpy was continuing the lessons for Chet that Samuel had not completed because of his relatively early death.

In those Oklahoma years, Patsy's principal task was taking care of the home and bringing up Diane and Deirdre. Nevertheless, she also found the time to reach out to the community and be active in the YWCA, a home for pregnant girls, her church, and also a social club. Chet says she developed her social connections and applied herself steadfastly to elaborating a clear role in community institutions and carving out her own niche. Furthermore, she did far more than her share of entertaining. He thinks she "manifested herself," which is a way of saying that while Patsy supported him and his independence, she also had a way of establishing her own identity and what she stood for, which didn't stop her from playing to the hilt the faculty wife role and having lots of other university people over. Of course, it was all helped by having a nice house, which had cost $18,000 in 1961. He thinks the house's layout and setting, with rosebushes, trees, and other features, made it a comfortable setting in which to receive friends. Their place also had a garage with an apartment that they rented to nurses.

I ask Chet about the couple's manner of reconciling their differences, and he makes it clear that in the domain of child-rearing, he deferred to Patsy. As a rule, he never argued with her or kicked up a fuss. He preferred to withdraw or go to sleep. He underlines once again his own personal approach to discord, emphasizing that he rarely if ever has to contend with feeling overwhelmingly angry. He even suggests I talk to Patsy about this, but he's confident he never shouts, and he has certainly never slapped his children. Indeed, he wonders if he was easily pushed around by the children. At any rate, the time they spent in the Oklahoma house was good. He points out that the two children did well in school, with Diane skipping a grade because of her impressive academic performance. Chet did his part by driving 17 miles each morning to take the children to the university school.

In the summer of 1965, Patsy had acute abdominal pain that necessitated surgery, revealing the diagnosis of an atypical appendicitis. Then, when given penicillin, she had an allergic reaction and almost died. Further complications set in that made her recovery long and arduous. Fortunately, her parents were visiting at the time and were able to stay to help Chet care for Diane and Deirdre while their mother struggled for her life. At that juncture, Chet had to confront some real questions that cause many of us to shudder, even at the mere thought of posing them hypothetically. He first considered whether the children should visit their mother, as she was hospitalized in such a precarious condition. His final decision was not to let them see her, fearing that it would be an unnecessarily traumatic experience for them and for her. Then he thought long and hard about what he would do if Patsy passed away and left him with the task of being a single parent. In his mind he opted to remain single and raise the children by himself, but he thanked his stars for not having to prove that he had the mettle to run a house without the help of a loving partner.

Experiences of this sort stop even the most stubborn of us in our tracks. Now, Chet sits in front of me reflecting on Patsy's possible demise and he concludes that it was a formative experience for everybody in the family. It was the second difficult medical problem for Patsy, and Chet thinks she emerged from it with clearly reduced vivaciousness and with a more pronounced soberness of spirit, although he doubts outsiders noted this change in her. Afterward, life was more precious to both of them, and Chet thanked the medical staff for their support and help and moved on with definite relief. But I stay temporarily riveted on this description of Chet's short-lived experience of watching his own wife dance with death. The commingled helplessness and fear must take a long time to get over, and that is without being directly the dance partner. I recognize full well, in today's parlance, that I have not been there and I have not done that. I do not know that experience, although I can hear my mother's Bajan reminder to keep me humble: "What en meet me en pass me."

We return then to the unfinished theme of life in Oklahoma, and I ask about his increasing recognition as a seasoned professional. Chet answers by talking about the fact that while at Oklahoma he was named a senior consultant to the Job Corps, Peace Corps, and Office of Employment Opportunity. He was also named to a number of national committees of the American Psychiatric Association, while developing increased access to local power structures such as the NAACP and the Urban League, ultimately becoming vice-president of both local chapters.

He was also still in Oklahoma when he first complained to a Black staff member of the National Institute of Mental Health about the lack of Blacks on NIMH committees. Then he discussed the complaint with a Los Angeles colleague and boyhood friend, Al Cannon, and the ideas about what they should do to force changes continued to germinate even after he left Oklahoma to go to Harvard.

Chet explains that his connection with the Peace Corps started after the Corps' chief psychiatrist, Joe English, heard Chet give a public lecture at a professional meeting. Chet's role as a senior consultant was to provide advice on certain research projects, help give exit interviews to volunteers who had completed their service, aid with the reentry problems of volunteers, help determine the job assignments of trainees, and participate in established in-country training. He maintains he has always been enthusiastic about the Peace Corps and considers it a great privilege to have participated in it. He also thinks the impact on the foreign countries and on the volunteers themselves was just fantastic. His activities with the group allowed him to see firsthand the capacity of humans to live in conditions of privation.

In significant contrast to Chet's obvious reticence in talking about money and in negotiating salaries, he was bold in approaching his chairman, Jolyon West, around 1965 to present the case for his promotion to the rank of full professor. Chet felt he met all the criteria relative to scholarly productivity, and he also thinks it was obvious he was an excellent chief of the biggest clinical service in the department. Unabashedly, he claimed the right to rapid promotion and was in fact rewarded. His superiors were also no doubt aware of his national standing and recognized that Chet was being repeatedly offered jobs at such places as Harvard, Meharry Medical College, Howard University, the University of Washington, the University of Southern California, and the University of Texas at Houston. Chet had also looked earlier at the chairmanship of the Department of Psychiatry at the University of the West Indies in Jamaica but thought the cultural contrasts would have been particularly difficult for his family.

Chet seems to have well worked out in his mind at the time the solid rationale for claiming early promotion, and it is clear that the issue was important to him. He goes on to note his definite popularity among the Arts and Sciences faculty at the University of Oklahoma, the fact that at the time the university was celebrating its founding, and that he had been invited to write an article to be included in the university's time vault that would be opened at its 150th anniversary. Chet had a high opinion of his own standing and notes that Jolyon West never gave him any idea of whether the promotion request would be hard to fulfill.

In an aside, Chet comments that West was a remarkable mentor who really enjoyed his role as "kingmaker." West enjoyed taking credit for being responsible for the success of underlings. Chet also underscores West's sense of honor and his serious commitment to his faculty's success. If West said he would do something, then he did it. He never promised what he couldn't deliver. If he remained silent, then he might not do it. Chet notes that West also might not tell you what he was planning to do; West loved the ritualistic pleasure of "bestowing" it on you. West apparently did not like the comparison, but Chet saw West as being very much like Ace, who always treated Chet like the little brother—with affection, but also without fearing Chet as a threat.

In 1967, West went on sabbatical to UCLA. At the same time, a former Harvard roommate wrote and asked Chet for recommendations of individuals who would be suitable for Alfred North Whitehead Fellowships tenable at Harvard's School of Education. The roommate subsequently wrote back and invited Chet to submit his own application, which was quickly accepted. West encouraged Chet to take his sabbatical year at Harvard, and even increased his salary so that the fellowship, in matching the salary, would provide more financial freedom during the year in Cambridge. So Chet and his family took off for Harvard, with the clear plan of returning to Oklahoma.

While Chet was away, however, West decided to stay at UCLA as head of the psychiatry department. He promptly invited Chet to join him there at the expiration of the fellowship year. Chet thought Los Angeles would be distracting, and he feared losing his high level of productivity, so he turned down West's offer. Then quickly came the joint offer from the School of Education and the Medical School that he stay at Harvard. He accepted it but rejected the additional suggestion that he become associate dean of the Medical School because he had no interest in an administrative position. (He in turn recommended that they consider Alvin

Poussaint, who was at the time on the faculty at Tufts University.) Chet cannot recall who first made the suggestion that he stay at Harvard, although he does vaguely remember holding discussions with the deans of the two relevant faculties. However, he does point out that lots of people knew of his presence at Harvard during the fellowship year, including well-placed professors such as Leon Eisenberg, with whom he taught a course for residents in psychiatry at the Massachusetts General Hospital. Also, Jack Ewalt had invited Chet several years before to come to Harvard to lead the psychiatry department at the Boston City Hospital.

It was at the beginning of this fellowship year at Harvard that a family member was diagnosed with a chronic illness that caused considerable sadness in the Pierce clan. It touches Chet, who consistently talks of the good fortune that he has had in life. He would like to give all his loved ones similar good fortune, but it will not be so. And he recalls with profound sadness how the family tried to protect him in the midst of it, when someone said at home, "We have to stop talking about this because it upsets Daddy." He thinks Patsy would accuse him of fleeing to work and denying it all, and he grants that she bore a heavier share of the burden. He is not happy about that, and once again to her credit she never showed any anger over this, which does not in turn diminish his guilt.

It remains important to Chet that Patsy would likely refer to him as an excellent father, although probably only a so-so husband. The lower grade in regard to their relationship he thinks is due mostly to the persistence of the traditional role relationships in his house. He was clearly not the man to volunteer to go to the store, although that would doubtless contrast with his readiness to adjust his schedule to fit the needs of his children. It is sobering, this business of grading your own family performance. However, a serious part of the age-seventy transition must be to issue the marks honestly. He grades Patsy as an excellent mother and wife and considers it the most robust proof of the magnificence of Providence.

While at the South Pole, Chet wrote a number of children's stories and special letters to Diane and Deirdre, who were very much on his mind. The six stories that follow are prime examples of what he wrote at the time. They accompanied gifts he sent to his daughters. He also wrote other stories, titled "The Peacock" and "The Horse." The stories speak for themselves, at once translating an unusually artistic side of Chet while also highlighting a powerful connection between father and children. I think the isolation must have evoked pleasant thoughts of attractive, innocent children. And I think readily of my own reaction to enforced separation from family, times when I conjure up my wife and children in tableaux of remarkable beauty.

5

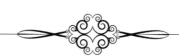

The Return to Cambridge

In 1968, Chet joined the Harvard School of Education as an Alfred North Whitehead Fellow, and his family and he rented an apartment located near Massachusetts General Hospital. When later he obtained a permanent Harvard professorial appointment, the family all moved to a house in Jamaica Plain, a racially and socioeconomically diverse Boston neighborhood known for its arboretum and pond. Patsy chose the house, a two-family dwelling located close to public transportation. In a division of roles that Chet and Patsy have developed over the years, she dealt with the realtors independently of Chet and settled on the type of building that would give her easy access to help because Chet was traveling a lot at the time. The house is smaller and less imposing than their Oklahoma home, but over time they have adjusted to its limitations. They currently live in the downstairs flat and also use the finished basement. In his own descriptive terminology, Chet finds it comfortable and satisfactory but certainly not elegant.

The house is owned by Patsy, a decision that was based on Chet's adhering to his father's early counsel and the later advice of his lawyers. There are, not surprisingly, other assets that he has kept in his own name. But he asserts a kind of righteous and moral justification for conceding ownership of this principal property to his wife. He says, "She deserves it," and I can hear the tenderness in his voice that suggests the legal decision may also have some emotional exculpatory basis. I think the emotion has to do with her deserving the house, given all she's put up with in the many years with Chet. I'm aware I may be hearing other voices besides Chet's on this topic, and I quickly realize why. Growing up in Barbados taught me cruel lessons about the different ways of "owning" property. In my Barbadian village, wives were joint owners of their homes with their husbands on moral, religious, and cultural—but not legal—grounds. However, I knew more than one woman who woke up one morning to find her house had been sold by one secret, unilateral action of the husband. And others, at the husband's death, found the house willed to someone else. It was a cruel hoax played on unsuspecting women by their bitter or angry husbands. But I learned that moral or cultural ownership of property had no standing in the eyes of the law. I am pleased, in an almost childish way, that the primary residence takes on special meaning for Chet.

He has never dreamt of having another house, and he points out that in general he and Patsy have lived very simply. Whatever extra money they possessed went to entertainment and travel, not to decorating the home. In fact, they have only one car, a 10-year-old Chevrolet Nova, that may soon need replacing. Chet doesn't look forward to buying a new car because he sees the interplay of today's automobile prices with the reality of changing from a salary to a pension, and he knows he will lose in the deal. Fortunately, Patsy and he don't drive much anymore, and the subway remains a reliable transportation method that suits their needs well.

The discussion of house and car takes us naturally to talk of clothes. As we know, Chet's father had clearly set a high standard of stylish dressing, and it's evident Samuel saw some of a man's worth reflected in the clothes worn by the individual. Chet even repeats what he has said before about his father's consistently elegant appearance and the father's readiness to give his sons advice about clothing and the stores to shop at. Chet, in contrast, sees himself as rumpled and points out that even if he starts out looking neatly attired in the morning, by afternoon he has once again taken on a rumpled look. Patsy has always thought he should dress better, and their daughters have often joined her in suggesting how he might, for example, improve the color coordination of his shirt, suit, and tie. At Oklahoma, Chet wore the traditional physician's white coat much of the time, which allowed him to sidestep the problem of wardrobe altogether. His return to Harvard offered him the chance of changing to a tweedy look, a stylistic standard that was surely below the one Samuel represented in Glen Cove society.

Chet adds that he never worried about what clothes meant. But that is perceptibly only half a truth, as he raises the concept of the work site culture and then goes on to explain that he never wanted to be seen as a cultural rebel, which he grants is easily exemplified by the clothes one wears. So, as he talks, it is obvious he has given considerable thought to what clothes mean. Indeed, he has reflected on the idea of dressing to avoid cultural incongruence and consciously finding a middle-of-the-road stance, one that neither identifies him as a revolutionary nor makes him appear to be "Roman," as opposed to being "like the Romans," which is Chet's preference. That is his way of talking guardedly about the task of adapting sartorially to mainstream institutions. It is an objective we both agree often befuddles some Black youth who want to follow their adolescent instincts but also desire acceptance from a conservative White organization. But, of course, Chet had had lots of practice in fitting clothes to the environment, without necessarily going overboard and becoming an elegant Samuel. I remind myself that this was a return to Harvard, a place where he'd already taken two degrees.

Chet finds another explanation for preferring the rumpled, nonelegant look and talks about being too big for a regular store and not big enough for the tall man's store. So he just settled over the years for going to the Harvard Coop. This is one time I laugh openly. My own stature makes Chet's struggle moderately amusing, because small men in America have often had to devise their own ingenious ways of finding reasonable clothes, although things are much better now than thirty years ago, when the offerings of every passable men's shop seemed to start around size 40. The other part of the joke is that facing the sartorial drought for small men in the States I turned to Europe and haven't looked back since then. Chet knows, too, that I am closer to Samuel in his practical approach to men's fashion than I am to Chet's, and I really guffaw when I consider my most recent visit to the Harvard Coop. I thought then they ought to fire the buyer who purchases their men's clothes. But the resulting change might disorient Chet unnecessarily.

After becoming serious again, I toy with the notion that like his fear of confronting his explosive potential around the race question, Chet sidesteps his unwillingness to put classy clothes on a body that he must know and has known for a long time is really imposingly attractive. Still, his claim of seeing no value in dressing, while being partly false, is also in a sense legitimate. He doesn't have to dress in order to establish his value, which is apparent both physically and psychologically. This rejection of a standard so important to his father also highlights Chet's clear emphasis on a pathway that relies less on money and the things money can buy. Even that is partly contradictory, as Chet well knows. His earlier arrival at Harvard's Lowell House as an undergraduate had been made possible by his father's attention to money and the senior Samuel's foresight in preparing for Chet's university education. Chet could reject money and clothes all he wanted, but it was Samuel's good fiscal sense that ultimately ensured he had the luxury to take on the tweedy Harvard look.

I daresay the fundamental question may ultimately be what's inside a suit. Chet's position on this may be admirably conservative, but Samuel was on to something that for many Blacks is hard to ignore. It is that an individual's clothes often evoke a reaction in an observer that can ultimately be either positive or negative. Putting on the right clothes can give an individual additional points in the competitive marketplace. Many Blacks can make good use of that extra edge.

As I expected, Chet isn't buying my point of view. Not at all. So I hazard a shot in the dark, anticipating the response before I frame the question. No, he does not have business cards, and he has never had any. I lecture him on the cultural symbolism of business cards and stationery. I even tell him the joke I heard 20 years ago, as I sought to join the Yale faculty, about a rationale for Yale's low salaries that included the right to use official Yale stationery for one's correspondence. The humorous point was that it was a terrific honor to have the privilege of using stationery with the royal blue Yale crest.

Chet doesn't join my joke with much enthusiasm, and he points out that he has consistently refused to join the ritual. By the time he got to Harvard, he had been teaching 16 years, had been on the faculties at Cincinnati and Oklahoma, and had used lots of different stationery. When he arrived at Harvard, he was presented with stationery and had never thought of making it up himself. He never felt disadvantaged or penalized by not having a card and thought it unseemly to walk around saying he was a professor at Harvard. He explains he didn't want to appear like a member of the nouveau riche; there was no class in that. He was always deliberately circumspect about telling anyone he was a teacher at Harvard.

Just to be a bit provocative, I mention a number of academics across the country who do their best to maximize their affiliations with prestigious institutions. I remind him of the "dream team" metaphor, so commonly employed now in sports, and its applicability to the academy where universities repeatedly advertise their capacity to recruit distinguished teachers. Chet insists he would never talk like that even if he thought it. He certainly appreciates the need in certain contexts to promote publicity, but it wouldn't be his style. It is too self-congratulatory, even if the facts are true. He finally utters the stinging comment that I hoped would not come so soon. He rejects the equivalence of status with things like business cards, suits, or cars and suggests that such trappings degrade the Black community. I think it a heavy burden to place on Black people as a group, even though I appreciate Chet's preference for quiet, compelling excellence, the type that speaks for itself. I point out that even exaggerated understatement, such as the tradition some university presidents have of using stationery with no street address, is a signal symbol that attracts attention, enhances identification, and obviously magnifies some White people's self-esteem. Blacks don't deserve to carry all the weight of Chet's criticism, and Chet has to know it. So I return to the rather elementary notion that, possessing the physical and psychological characteristics that speak so elegantly on his behalf, Chet can afford to be cavalierly dismissive of aesthetic rituals. However, even that is inexact, because Chet loves manners. The task is to define his conception of it, which you see, if observant enough, in his graceful personal interactions, his gently sophisticated turn of a written or spoken word, his insistence on deferential service to women, and his tenacious public respect for members of the Black group.

During his sabbatical year at Harvard in 1968, Chet had no specific obligations, so he designed his own schedule. He functioned as an attending psychiatrist in a clinic at Massachusetts General Hospital, where he taught residents in psychiatry. Chet also took a course in demography at Harvard because he thought it important that Blacks understand how people and populations moved and changed. This was a longstanding interest of his, one he had nurtured somewhat during a tutorial he took with an anthropologist named Bill Biddle at Oklahoma. Chet had become interested in the history of all-Black towns that were located especially in Oklahoma, Kansas, and Colorado. Because of its geographic proximity, the Oklahoma enclave of Boley attracted his attention. Chet explains that Boley was set up just after the Civil War because two White men had a bet about whether Blacks could build and run a town. Boley had substantial economic success and political stability, and some of its families acquired considerable wealth. Over the years, however, it clearly declined; and when Chet got to see it, he thought it represented definite decrepitude. Chet still enjoyed the experience and thought it worthwhile to confirm that Blacks could organize and be effective even under difficult circumstances. However, he was not able, in his study of Boley, to grasp fully what forces drove some of the town's citizens to attempt a movement back to Africa in the 1920s. Apparently, a significant part of the town's wealth was dissipated in that endeavor.

Chet's third area of focus during that first academic year was on developing his idea of a Black children's domestic exchange. At the time, he had heard that airplanes were running about 25% empty. So he thought it would be a great learning experience to take a child with him

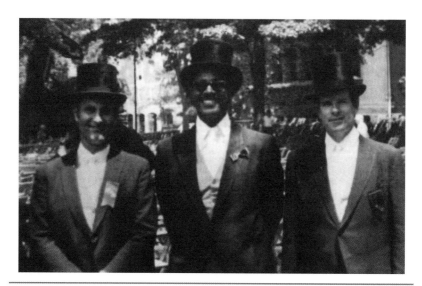

Harvard commencement marshals *(left to right)* Ed Davis, Chester Pierce, and John Watkins, circa 1968.

if, for example, he was traveling to San Francisco. Once there, he could hand the child over to someone who would act as the child's caregiver; in the meantime, a judge, for example, would volunteer to have the child sit as observer in his court for a day. Chet would then take the child back on the return trip to their departure point. Chet explains that the concept grew out of two of his own experiences. The first was linked to the time he was studying the Tarahumara Indians in Mexico, when he took one of their children with him on her first trip outside the region to see the city of Chihuahua. It was the child's baptismal confrontation with modern technology. The second formative experience found Chet at a New York City party on Central Park South. The Black men in the room were all well off, influential, and well placed professionally and politically. Chet decided at the time that Black youth, by age 15, should have the opportunity to be present at a party like that and see that class of Black male.

Chet took the idea of this domestic children's program to Frank Williams, a famous civil rights lawyer and former United States ambassador to the United Nations. Apparently, Williams, who was then at Columbia University, liked the proposal, thought it had political appeal, and went so far as to pull together a group of eminent individuals to discuss it. At the meeting, a distinguished psychologist, whom Chet preferred to leave unnamed, opposed the concept, and Williams let it drop because he obviously felt it important to have unanimous support.

Chet was confounded by the psychologist's opposition; Chet had even considered the international implications of the concept, saying enthusiastically and with a flash of light in his eyes, "Imagine a 12-year-old spending time in Afghanistan." Of course, Chet has no trouble at all acknowledging that times have changed, and many people would now be concerned about putting young children in the care of adults who are not well known to the guardians of the children.

Chet talks more about the psychologist, a man I have heard a lot about but have never met. Some years after the children's exchange meeting, the same psychologist was on a program with Chet at Boston University and once again attacked Chet's ideas and presentation. Chet reports that some onlookers were surprised that he took the criticism gracefully and did not fight back. Chet makes a point I've heard before: When Blacks argue in front of Whites, potentially dangerous information is given freely to Whites, and Chet won't engage in that activity. He believes Blacks can and should resolve their differences in their own deliberations.

I am bothered by that explanation, and I point out to Chet that I was witness some years ago to his participation on a panel with other Black professionals at a meeting where the audience was entirely Black. Chet and another panelist clearly disagreed, but Chet obstinately refused to defend himself. I recalled the occasion quite well because a friend and I had actually chatted about Chet's refusal to respond to his colleague's critique. So it is not just the presence of Whites that can make Chet bite his tongue and remain silent. Chet argues that he likes his ideas, once expressed, to speak for themselves and he also doesn't like the spectacle of participating in public contests.

At a recent conference, Chet and I were participants in a symposium and I reminded him that I had challenged him on an idea that we were discussing. But he ducked my intellectual provocation. Chet comments that on this score he and I are different. He thinks I enjoy the process of resolving a philosophical dilemma or arguing out a point. But he prefers throwing an idea out and then having the intellectual community kick it around and do with it what they will. In contrast, he dislikes putting forward some notion and subsequently promoting it or trying to impose it on others.

It is doubtless a quaint way to think about having an impact on public policy, being so deliberately reticent and nonargumentative about one's positions. It's troubling, because I know Chet has spent a lot of his life forging an impact on organizations, and I find it hard to digest this particular point. I bring it up again, and I ask what is really the worst thing that could happen if he publicly argued out his ideas. He hesitantly suggests there might be, in our case, some potential for his carrying a grudge against me as a result of a caustic interaction. He raises, too, the inappropriateness of breaching boundaries of civility and points out that often in these intellectual contexts the combatants are more disputatious than really interested in the inherent worth of their ideas.

I circumnavigate that point and, with my mind on the Dallas airport incident, ask him why he is so afraid of his own anger. He says as a child he was afraid of being angry, and he partly relates it to the disparity in size between him and others his own age. He recognized quite early that children around him were in reality defenseless if he exercised his own physical capability to do harm to them. As a marker of his imposing size, he wore long pants instead of knickers when he was a cub scout. Then Chet moves to an incident that occurred when he was in high school. An assistant football coach told him to leave his feet to carry out a block on an opponent. In the practice session, Chet did just that, and another coach bawled him out for leaving his feet. Chet went over to the second coach, obviously intent on beating him, but teammates grabbed Chet and prevented the impending explosion. Chet was "sobered" by the realization of what he had almost done and appreciated the implications of his potential for "terrible wrath."

There is no question that Chet is lucky. He managed to escape paying the price for learning about his anger. I think back to the time when I was in the Army and a sergeant who had picked on me mercilessly for months came up to me and asked me where I had just come from. I told him I wouldn't answer his question, and I walked off. His interrogation served no purpose, and it came after repeated incidents of his attempting to persecute me and break my spirit. I was angry, seeing blue and red and all the other colors that usually spell tragedy. There's no question that I was insubordinate in not giving a direct and polite response to the sergeant's inquiry. But somewhere inside, I knew I had to walk off or end up doing something that would certainly have taken me directly to the stockade.

I tell Chet there must be some middle ground. There has to be room for what I call effective aggression because we both know it makes no sense to be repeatedly trampled on. Chet concedes there comes a time when one has to stand up and defend himself. The central problem is trying to figure out what's worth a major argument or fight. For him, the academic symposium is not a place for getting combative. It's only words. While academics argue, serious decisions are being made that affect people's lives. In that practical context, where people's lives are at stake, Chet thinks it is worthwhile being aggressive, but not in the marketplace of a panel or symposium where the audience won't even think about the ideas a few hours later. He also cautions about the toll that anger takes on everybody and suggests that an episode of belligerence is often precipitated because a particular individual is trying to build a wall all by himself. He thinks it wise just to put a brick into the structure and let others do their part. Chet insists this is not to be taken as his meaning that defending oneself is unimportant.

I want to be sure, nevertheless, that I understand fully this aspect of Chet's thesis, so I ask again why he recoils from public argument with Black colleagues. I tell Chet he can't deny that he manipulates language effectively; consequently, in many of these discussions he would easily carry the day, given his cleverness at formulating a position and reasoning logically. Chet's reply stuns me for a second. It's arrogance that keeps him out of so many of these arguments with Blacks. He also adds that in some of these exchanges with colleagues, he has the feeling that some Black men are persuaded they have to get the better of him. Chet feels compelled to avoid that kind of fray, that sort of contest. He then makes a lateral shift to mention another subgroup of Black men who are frightened off once they hear his credentials. As a teacher, he worries about Black men who flee him. Chet sees these Black males as amorphous and ambivalently occupying the intellectual scene. He is always upset when he can't do something to calm their fears. He talks specifically about some of his African American students who have difficulty framing their needs and then contending with them in a mature fashion.

The Boston University experience with the psychologist is more substantive than it may at first appear. On the one hand, it is related to the problem of Black men and women trying to work out their struggles in front of Whites. On the other hand, the presence of Whites can be seen as irrelevant and unrelated to the issue of Blacks having to resolve the difficulties they have with each other. Black-on-Black disputes are particularly painful to Black intellectuals, but expecting only solace and friendship from one's Black colleagues is a wasted dream. This is a painful lesson I have learned along the way at several points, and it is a subject Chet and I spend time on repeatedly at our many lunches in the Harvard Square restaurants when I drive up to see him on Fridays. I point out, for example, that Black liberals like myself like to pretend there are no Black conservatives. But simple common sense tells me there must be Blacks, too, who wish to destroy affirmative action, however it is defined. Somehow, Black intellectuals prefer the myth that there is total homogeneity in Black thought. It is comforting for us to believe that 20 million other Black people really agree with our sense of reality. I recall stating my opinion about some issue related to the rearing of Black children at a meeting of mental health professionals one day in New York. After I had finished, a psychologist told me he had discussed the same issue with James Comer, a well-known colleague of mine at Yale, and Comer's view was different from mine. How could two Black psychiatrists have opposing ideas about the same subject? I held my tongue respectfully at the time. But I realized later that even the general public doesn't like to think of Black intellectuals differing among themselves. Still, as Blacks acquire experience, technical knowledge, and wide exposure to different cultural values, their ensuing thought processes are bound to cover a wide spectrum that will lead the Black individuals themselves to end up in vastly different camps.

This does not budge Chet from another basic point he is intent on framing. He argues that as a manifestation of the ubiquity and omnipresence of racism in the United States, Whites automatically and instinctively use even minor discord by Blacks to promote divisiveness, doubt, and strife. Blacks become trained to "overexpose" themselves and their plans in the service of comforting Whites. In turn, this facilitates Whites' efforts to manipulate Blacks. It often further leads to verification of the defeated or inferior status of Blacks. Chet insists that he has confirmed Blacks' tendency to overexpose gratuitously in the presence of Whites through empirical research he has carried out with colleagues.

We pick up the thread of Chet's return to Cambridge and review his basic activities in 1969, when he would have completed the fellowship year and formally been named to his faculty post. The Medical School paid two-thirds of his salary for his teaching of medical students and participation in committee work; the School of Education paid for about a third of his time, which he allocated to lecturing in three courses a year, and also provided him an office and secretarial support. Chet earned an additional small part of his salary from supervising psychiatry residents who were in training at Massachusetts General Hospital, one of Harvard's teaching facilities, and served on some of its hospital committees. The dean of the Medical School arranged for Chet to see patients at the Massachusetts Institute of Technology's health service. Service at MIT contributed to part of his salary, but it also suited his travel schedule because most other consultative activities would generally have required him to be present at fixed times. In some years, Chet also taught at Harvard's School of Public Health, conducting seminars on international behavioral science or disaster management.

At various points in our dialogue, Chet has explained how these commitments in the context of work really added up to a comparatively small amount of time and ultimately to a correspondingly minimal amount of energy. Furthermore, no one ever dictated what he taught. With genuine amusement, he points out that he had no idea what a psychiatrist did in a school of education. So he simply set about to develop his own courses on topics such as propaganda, extreme environments, and sports and society.

Central to his negotiated activities in returning to Harvard was the compulsive wish to maximize control of his own time and thereby control of his energy. For those two elements, he clearly gave up any corresponding focus on money. Chet's insistent and consistent emphasis on time and his wish to control it as best he could highlights in my mind the tableau of a Black man's remaining independent in the bowels of a predominantly White organization like Harvard. Chet defined freedom in a way that makes most Blacks I know embarrassingly unfree.

Before his return to Harvard, Chet was invited to participate in planning sessions for the new television program *Sesame Street*, whose producers somehow knew of Chet's interest in children's stories. Joan Cooney, the driving force behind *Sesame Street*, invited community people, academics of all sorts, and artists to discuss topics such as what children should know about the grammatical use of prepositions. The program staff would listen attentively to the discussion before drawing up their own plan on how to implement the ideas on the show. Chet enjoyed these meetings, had lunch often with Cooney, and became a general consultant to *Sesame Street*. Chet and Cooney had discussed the impact of the television medium on children, which was not far from his more general interest in the broader topics of propaganda and brainwashing. Of course, Joan Cooney had been developing her own idealistic agenda of helping Black children. Chet pointed out that she noted how children were glued to television and she wanted to seize their interest to teach them through use of the medium to which they were already connected. So both Cooney and Chet were intrigued by the task of connecting to what held the children's interest by linking television to some pedagogical function. Chet saw Cooney as a White woman with very liberal interests; he noted that although filled with good intentions, she encountered difficulties in trying to push Blacks upward in her own organization. Chet recognized that having a progressive idea was one thing; implementing it in a problematic racial climate was quite another. In broader terms, the experience with Cooney at the Children's Television Workshop helped Chet conceptualize more clearly his thinking about children and about television and its portrayal of images and other visual content.

As I noted in Chapter 4, Chet had written a number of children's stories, particularly during his stay in Antarctica, that had never been published. One of them, "The Shell Fairy," was composed for his own children—and partly to console his brother's children because Burton had recently lost his wife in an unfortunate accident. In this story, Uncle Ishke is a gruff old sailor who loves children and adores telling them tales about his experiences all over the world. When Ishke plays his flute, it transfixes humans so they can understand certain experiences and emotions. Ultimately, Ishke becomes a fairy and disappears. But he leaves behind him a remarkable blessing for children. Whenever they put their ears to a seashell, they can have experiences and emotions that are particularly exotic and pleasant because of what they can hear emanating from the shell. The magic allows them, for example, to imagine and know how the sun rises over Dar es Salaam. One of Chet's friends, a Black composer and musician named T.J. Anderson, composed an operetta based on "The Shell Fairy" that Chet knows will be performed someday. Sara Beattie, a Black novelist, wrote the libretto. Hearing Chet talk about creatively communicating with children permits me a glimpse of his special tenderness, to which one does not have ready access. But I link this discussion about children's stories to an interaction I witnessed between him and his niece one day in his office and I realize that Chet is truly enamored of children and youth.

Before continuing with this line, however, I return to the subject of Chet's involvement in other media studies, particularly his observations about the portrayal of Blacks on television. One intriguing project was his study of television advertisements, in which he noted the following: Blacks talked little, and they had minimal contact with children; Whites reinforced their connection to families, but this was rarely done for Blacks; Blacks were shown eating but rarely talking; Whites were portrayed with profound depth behind them, Blacks with little or no space, which gave the impression that Whites controlled significantly more space than did Blacks; Whites never seemed to work, even though they controlled their resources, while Blacks sometimes worked but were never in control of resources.

These findings are worth considering in conjunction with those from another of Chet's early projects in which he examined television program content and focused on the way Blacks and Whites were portrayed solving problems. Whites sought their solutions by being reflective and in control of technology. Blacks solved their problems through confrontational and ineffective violence. The findings from these two studies demonstrated that television, as a popular communication medium in the Black and White communities, characterized Blacks differently from Whites. It is easy to see, too, in Chet's terms, that children looking at these images day after day would eventually internalize general principles about Blacks that would lead to a limited view and belief about what Blacks were capable of accomplishing in the world dominated by Whites. Chet's findings made it easier for me to understand why some Blacks had trouble believing that the lead characters in *The Cosby Show*, a doctor and a lawyer, were realistic. They struggled unsuccessfully with the notion that a Black family could actually control the kind of resources that the Huxtable family were portrayed as having.

Chet's observations about television led him to the powerful notion that children were more oppressed than minorities. It persuaded him that as a society, we enjoy succumbing to the myth that we are child-oriented and child-loving. Chet recounts an episode that was at the heart of a fascinating 1975 article on the topic of childism. He was waiting for a friend in the lobby of a New York hotel when he noticed that a woman turned to a child and said, "Honey, hand me that cigarette lighter, please." Chet points out that the White woman had a choice of two minorities (Chet and the child) and chose the child to "oppress." He underlines the importance of the choice and characterizes it as a form of violence, linking it also to what he sees as our poor regard for other species, or speciesism.

Chet deconstructs the tableau of the woman oppressing the child. First, she controlled the child's space. The child had to travel some distance to reach the lighter and therefore abandoned where she wanted to be and put herself in the service of comforting and nurturing the grown woman. The child's use of space was defined and limited by the adult. Second, the child donated time to meet the woman's needs. Third, the child's mobility was put at the service and comfort of the woman, who in turn was conserving her own life force. Finally, the child's energy, necessary for the implementation of mobility, was put at the service of the oppressor. Chet points out that these four elements are commonly intertwined in the interest of oppression, and the oppressor is the one with control over the four factors. The degree to which one controls the elements in any given context can provide a useful quantitative assessment of the degree of oppression. Chet further argues that in a general sense in any oppressive context, one's degree of personal stress increases the more one cedes control of the elements. One can decrease the stress by correspondingly asserting greater control over the four factors. Sometimes one attempts to do so through retaliatory violence. Furthermore, persistent maintenance of a high level of stress can lead to substantive hopelessness and helplessness. Chet feels this explanatory model not only provides us an insight into oppression but also helps us to understand retaliatory violence better.

I have no trouble at all applying the model to one of the most obvious contexts of oppression, the period of basic training that all military recruits must endure before they are welcomed by their peers into the brotherhood of macho men. Before they cross the magical threshold, however, these young civilians coming directly off the street have to endure severe limitations on their space, time, energy, and mobility so they will eventually appreciate who owns their minds and bodies. I suspect its tolerance by society has to do with its being a tradition long made honorable over the years and by the complex reality of raising standing armies.

The recognition of what most of us do to our children makes me blanch, however, and I am made no calmer by Chet's increasing my awareness of the techniques used by us all to subjugate each other. It is also clearer to me why Chet, and I, find it hard to accept the rituals of psychoanalysis. Turn it any way you wish, at the heart of the analysis is the analyst's insistence on controlling the patient's time, space, and mobility. This will easily be labeled by those devoted to the art as a simplistic distortion. But make the analyst White and the patient Black, and you have lots of terrain for misunderstanding about dominance, control, and oppression in the treatment context, which in my experience is much more than the Black patient need take responsibility for.

It is easy to see that all this preoccupation with children is not just a theoretical exercise for Chet, and I ask about his own children and their activities in the period after he had joined the Harvard faculty. Diane had been to a private school called Brimmer and May and then moved around 1970 to Hampshire College, whose unconventional system she liked. Chet recalls no formal discussion with her about her choice of college, although he acknowledges the clear expectation that she continue her education. He had a permissive style about those things, founded partly on the experience with his own mother, who had confidence in him and never tried to prescribe or influence his decisions of that ilk. Besides, he explains with some obvious smugness, Diane's grades were very good and she could have gone wherever she wished. So he was relaxed about her choice of college, noting that she was caught up in the spirit of the time and influenced also by Hampshire's membership in the five-college consortium with Smith, Amherst, University of Massachusetts, and Mount Holyoke. Diane later completed her master's degree in communications at the University of Hawaii and her law degree at Harvard.

Deirdre, being younger, continued at Brimmer and May for 2 more years. She eventually transferred to the Palfrey School, pursuing a strong interest in drama. When time came to apply to college, she preferred to stay close to home. She was accepted by a number of colleges and finally chose Emerson College because of its emphasis on theater and communications. After Deirdre's freshman year, Chet proposed that she take a trip around the world, a gift he talks about with more tenderness than I have ever seen in him. He met with her for a year to plan the trip, which took about 3 months. She did it alone, and it turned out to be a critical experience for her. On her return, she completed the 2 remaining years of college with honor grades. At her graduation, she had no wish to attend graduate school immediately. But now he worries about her taking care of herself without a graduate degree.

As a father myself, I cringe at the obvious mélange of pain and love in Chet's discussion of his daughters, and I hope to do justice to his emotions as I relate this aspect of the dialogue. He certainly does not describe his two children in quite the same tone, and there are differing levels and qualities of concern for each of them. It is the unrelenting burden of the father who loves his children so much that he would love to absorb all their suffering for them, even though he knows that nature will not permit it. Each generation must hack its own way through the forest, without direct assistance from those who have gone before. Parents can purchase the machete and even pay for the instruction in its use, but the child will wield it on her own. Chet knows it, and the limitation on his ability to grant more help to his children sticks uncomfortably and indigestibly in his throat.

Patsy took advantage of the daughters' maturing and moving out to live on their own. She enrolled at Boston University and completed another master's degree, this one in social work, around 1978. Then she went to work at a local mental health center. Chet takes on a look of contentment as he describes how they were able to increase the chances of traveling together once the child-rearing task was out of the way. Their relationship continued to be good in his eyes; they laughed a lot, and she maintained her stance that was so uncritical and supportive of him. He relied unceasingly on the fact that he found her smarter than he and certainly a better judge of people and situations.

As the 1960s came to a close and transitioned inexorably into the 1970s, the country was in considerable racial turmoil, and every major institution was being reexamined in light of newly defined relationships between Blacks and Whites. This was true also for American psychiatry. It was, in 1968, a signal experience when a staff member from the National Institute of Mental Health (NIMH) tutored Chet about all the money the NIMH controlled and the correspondingly small impact that Blacks had on how and where that money was spent. Chet's ensuing discussion with Al Cannon, a militant Black psychiatrist from UCLA, led to their joint formulation of the idea that Black psychiatrists needed to have greater influence on the major organizations that controlled what happened in the psychiatry arena. Those organizations were the NIMH, with a major budget used to fund research, new service initiatives, and training of mental health professionals; the American Psychiatric Association (APA), a professional group that had substantial impact on the national practice of psychiatry; and the American Board of Psychiatry and Neurology (ABPN), which controlled through an examination process the awarding of credentials to those qualified as specialist psychiatrists.

Chet points out that at the time, many Black psychiatrists were not even members of the APA; fewer had ABPN qualifications, and probably only a handful had participated on NIMH committees. As a result, APA leadership, for example, didn't even think about Blacks and their interests. Chet and Al Cannon developed the idea of a mechanism that could serve to focus pressure on these main groups and lead to changes in their way of organizationally conceptualizing Black interests. Chet and Cannon saw the value of forming the Black Psychiatrists of America (BPA), which was a symbolic protest against the APA. Not surprisingly, however, Chet did not advocate abandoning membership in the APA—he wished to have his cake and eat it too. He wanted the capacity to influence these organizations from within and without. Chet knew Blacks had to accomplish some change within the APA in order to influence the NIMH, journal editorial boards, the ABPN, and so on.

Chet further exercised leadership by writing John Gardner, a former Secretary of the Department of Health, Education, and Welfare, seeking advice on how to bring about change in the NIMH. Gardner moved to help, and a delegation from the NIMH went to Harvard to hear the complaints of a group of Black psychiatrists organized by Chet. Out of these discussions ultimately came the decision that a special minority section should be established within the NIMH that would oversee the allocation of money to researchers working on minority interests and to the training and education of future minority mental health clinicians and researchers.

Having made progress in starting discussions with the prestigious NIMH, Chet and Al Cannon organized a group of Black psychiatrists to confront the APA at their annual meeting in 1969 and demand that the APA be more cognizant of the needs and interests of Black psychiatrists who were members of the organization. This certainly led eventually to changes in structure and governance within the APA, but it also resulted in the establishment of the BPA as a professional society that has maintained its viability to this day. The BPA celebrated its twenty-fifth anniversary at a national meeting in New York City in 1994, and it marked its 1996 convention with a well-publicized gala on the African continent, in Senegal.

Chet was therefore at the very center of things when Black psychiatrists agitated for greater influence in the affairs of organized American psychiatry. As a result, more Blacks were appointed to APA committees; a Black was elected to the vice-presidency of the organization; a Black psychiatrist was hired to manage a minority affairs office within the APA; Blacks also gained broader representation on NIMH committees; and Chet was named to the ABPN board of directors after another Black psychiatrist turned down the original offer. A minority center was started at the NIMH, and Chet chaired its first study section. These were all impressive accomplishments. Yet Chet gave up leadership of the BPA in 1970, after a single year. He insists he always said he would do it for only a year. Not only did the activity take a lot of time, but support from the Black members was not resolutely strong, particularly because many of them did not follow through on their assignments. And he felt limited by his incapacity to galvanize the others to complete their tasks. He even feels the executive group gave good counsel but were slow to do more than that. So he thought others were more likely than he to be more successful in getting the organization to move.

This is the first time that Chet and I have ever discussed the BPA. But my own pain, endured during the 2 years I served as the BPA's president from 1982 to 1984, makes me doubtful that Chet's decision to renounce the leadership of the organization after such a brief time was done on the basis of simple administrative logic. When my disbelief shows clearly on my face, Chet goes on to amplify his explanation. He acknowledges that at the time he was confident no one would step forward to work harder than he was already working. At the same time, he worried that if he stayed on longer as leader, the group's resentment toward him would build. I wonder then whether he just wished to run away from the potential conflict. He articulates the idea that some people probably wanted to curb his excessive influence on the organization, and he suggests that the lack of cooperation he experienced was a form of passive resentment. In addition, he was at the same time being held responsible for everything related to the BPA, which in turn made him worry that the organization was not democratic enough, thereby blunting the growth of creativity in the BPA.

I dig deeper to uncover this sense of Chet's loneliness as BPA's president. He feels he worked hard and was effective, but he didn't feel "popular." I am wary of such terminology, although I think I understand what he means. But he has no difficulty in adding some longitudinal depth to his adjective. Even as a child he was popular, and during his stay in Oklahoma he exercised considerable leadership and could feel the high regard of those around him. In contrast, the BPA did not "receive" him, and he did not feel "endorsed." The image springs to mind of my being labeled a European Black by some of my detractors in the BPA, and I ask Chet if there was ever any concern about his lack of militancy or about his willingness to seek compromise with Whites. Chet denies that these issues could have been a problem for him because at the time the only person who could conceivably have claimed more militant credentials or spouted a more radical Black philosophy than he was Al Cannon, his boyhood friend from Long Island.

The circumstances in which Chet and I led the BPA seem different. But there is remarkable similarity in our disappointment at not having made an effective connection to all our constituents. It was an important lesson for me to digest—that leadership of a Black group is not carried off simply by force of intellect or by being eloquent about ideas whose merit is obvious. The Black group's insecurities must be handled adroitly and their strengths assiduously courted. Just because you are good for the group doesn't mean the group thinks you are good for them. And you cannot lead the Black group by ignoring the spectrum of individual Black political orientations represented within the system. The BPA experience represents a theme that deserves more reflection. And for both Chet and me, it symbolizes a discrepancy in our history of more successful leadership stints, particularly in predominantly White organizations.

An example of Chet's impressive success with other organizations is his sustained connection to the Polar Research Board (PRB), a component of the National Research Council that was established by the National Academy of Sciences in 1916. Chet was appointed to the PRB in 1968 and subsequently served several terms on it. He thinks his initial appointment to it resulted from his work in the Antarctic. However, American interest in polar studies eventually shifted more to the Arctic, with a focus on military, political, and economic issues. The PRB then was asked to turn its attention also to research issues raised by the renewed spotlight being shed on the Arctic, and Chet visited the Arctic region well over 20 times because of his scholarly preoccupation with extreme environments. Chet's polar work also included two terms as an adviser at the National Science Foundation's Division of Polar Programs. In addition, he served as an advisor to the U.S. Arctic Research Commission.

I ask what an average trip to the Arctic would be like. He offers the example of the PRB's receiving a request to study whether a larger part of Alaska should be opened to oil exploration. This would lead to a narrower question about the scientific implications of building a pipeline in the area. The PRB would then ask a team of six experts to visit Alaska and examine the engineering, ecological, and biological consequences of constructing the pipeline, while thinking about the possible human and animal responses to the environmental changes. Chet thinks most of these studies were done with an emphasis on science for the sake of science, especially with an eye to clarifying what happens to people in extreme conditions. But over the years, there has been increasing interest in the applicability of observations on extreme environments to analogous conditions, such as those existing in a spacecraft. Chet's own theoretical idea, however, is that what has been learned in the extreme exotic environments of the polar areas and space should be applicable to the extreme mundane environment of, for example, the ghetto areas of our cities.

Struck by the terminology, I ask for further clarification of these concepts. Chet explains that examples of extreme exotic environments are a submarine, a space vehicle, an undersea laboratory, or a polar desert. Civilian prisons, nursery schools for the very young, mental hospitals, and urban ghettos are examples of extreme mundane environments. Chet is at his maximum fluency, and it is clear he enjoys giving this lecture as much as I like hearing it. The stress an individual experiences in an extreme environment is inversely related to the support he experiences. Furthermore, even if support is given, it must be provided with consistency, reliability, and in a manner that is not rejecting. For example, the grudging provision of a welfare check is rejecting. So the tone of the support is also important. Chet makes clear that the chief enemy in all this is hopelessness. There are common pathways to diluting the stress of an extreme environment. Individuals must maximize their own control of space, time, mobility, and energy. They must take decisive and independent action to help themselves, and their supporters must provide group cohesion and compatibility in carrying out the task, which must also be clearly defined. Positive feedback for what one is doing also helps, as does knowledge that the length of time being spent in the extreme environment is limited. Chet emphasizes that training to perform tasks in the particular environment is a clear advantage, whereas amorphous structure and indefinite stays in the environment do not help.

Chet provides examples that elucidate these principles more fully. The more we know about the proposed extreme environment, the better we perform. That is the logical reason for carrying out fire drills. Prior knowledge also attenuates the tendency to be surprised. Surprise increases stress. Anticipating hostility and frailty from members of your own group helps, and prisoners of war should expect such behavior from one of their own. People who do well under stress have strong convictions. They tend to have greater trust in institutions to which they maintain an intellectual and affective connection. The fear of abandonment is crucial, and it speaks for strong emphasis on support. Being preoccupied by the stressor is, to a certain point, helpful. For example, focusing on the weather in the polar regions reduces the chance of being surprised by the unexpected arrival of a storm. On the other hand, one cannot be hypervigilant because hypervigilance uses up too much energy.

In summary, then, the extreme environment can be characterized by forced socialization, depression, spatial isolation, time elasticity, biological and sociological dysrhythmia, increased free time, noise extremes, loneliness, fear of abandonment, anxiety, panic, information fractionalization, boredom, and the inability to escape.

In a 1975 article, Chet makes the point that in comparing the exotic and mundane environments, "it is much more difficult in terms of psychological and physiological adjustment to be a ten-year-old inhabitant of Harlem than it is to be a forty-year-old aquanaut or astronaut." Chet felt that the societal support and commitment to the safety of the astronaut vastly outweighed any support the Harlem youngster could ever dream of having. Similarly, there remains great difference in the resources expended to support astronauts and eventually to reward their success, in contrast to what would support or reward the Black Harlemite.

I turn Chet to the extreme, mundane, environmental experience of the Black person trying to make it in the predominantly White institution, and I ask him how Black people can differentiate between the circumstance requiring vigilance and hypervigilance. Chet thinks it crucial for Blacks to recognize that they are alternatively under hypersurveillance and hyposurveillance. For example, in the work context, a Black male is regularly under hypersurveillance regarding what he does with White women. In the same employment context, no one may care how the Black maintenance man dresses. Chet reasons that it takes technique to differentiate between the two situations, to figure out what is at stake, and to be clear about the steps open to be taken. But he also is of the opinion that both Blacks and Whites can teach about these techniques, which are so important because they relate directly to the daily use of energy to protect oneself against racist aggressions.

Chet knows I am intrigued by whether he thinks both Blacks and Whites can teach these coping techniques. The question is central to my intellectual position in the debate about transracial adoptions. The cultural position taken by those who are against such adoptions is based on the claim that Black children need to be taught skills to cope with racist America, and only Blacks can teach such skills. I have labeled the claim political cant because I see nothing that makes Blacks uniquely placed to pass on a particular coping style to Black children, even if we could all agree on the particular ingredients that characterize the particular style.

Chet does know, however, some of the traits to which he refers. For example, he insists Blacks need to be taught how to be selectively silent in front of Whites as well as how to laugh in front of Whites because laughter sometimes suggests that the Black individual is not serious. Chet astounds me with the degree of thought he has put into this, and he continues quite seriously as he states that when a Black person laughs in front of Whites, he must be thoughtful and intentional. Chet warns against doing things that "verify your inferiority" and that confirm Whites' expectations that Blacks be "compatible, accepting, and of good cheer." Chet underlines his belief that we can teach and train people how to go into the extreme exotic environment, so it should be equally possible to prepare individuals for the extreme mundane context. But we both know it is a matter of societal will, and mundane environments do not captivate the imagination with the same compelling force as do exotic environments. Hence, the public purse opens to one and remains relatively closed to the other.

Chet's established interest in extreme environments also permitted formation of a nexus with his other well-defined preoccupation with sports. It is in this context that he and colleagues carried out comparative studies of the Mexican Tarahumara kickball race, conducted over a 250-mile distance at altitudes over 6,000 feet, and the Alaskan Iditarod, a dogsled competition traversing 1,049 miles between Anchorage and Nome. The researchers were interested in exploring "the limits of human endurance and the application of extreme motivation." In the kickball competition, a team of two to six players take turns kicking a small wooden ball around a circular course of 25 miles, and all team members must complete the entire race. In the Iditarod, the human racers, or mushers, must contend with extreme cold and limited sleep and take good care of their dogs. Chet and his colleagues compared the two races on the basis of use of space, fiscal resources, amount of gear, practice preparation, risk during the race, and other variables. The two races obviously had similarities and differences. But the researchers' comparative observations about these events afforded them broader speculation about the place of sport in society, particularly as to how games at that level of skill may not only provide entertainment. Such games also may permit the societal group to sharpen skills that relate to their continued survival and that promote religious or secular socialization.

In reviewing the parameters of Chet's return to Harvard, I recognize that I had arbitrarily decided to divide his 28 Harvard professorial years in half, which would extend this chapter from 1968 to 1982, the year he reached age 55, a year older than his biographical chronicler. He reminds me too that he wrote "Birthday Thoughts" in 1982, when he was probably in Nome, Alaska, watching the end of the Iditarod. It was in this extreme setting that Chet celebrated his birthday and contemplated his achievements. He can't remember the name of the famous Russian novelist who dubbed age 55 as awful, but he recalls that in 1982 he had the distinct feeling that he had had good fortune and a beautiful life.

He acknowledges that at 55 he had no administrative responsibility or pressure. He never wanted it. He never had the desire. He prized mainly the lack of obligation. By then, he had passed up the main administrative opportunities. He had been interviewed for chairmanships and deanships and had declined them all. He had also rejected the opportunity to express an interest in sub-cabinet-level jobs in Washington, D.C. He adds, "There is some blessing to anonymity."

Patsy had never even raised the issue of what he might do, whether he should change jobs, or whether he had accomplished enough. He uses a curious expression: "My life had plateaued." I ask whether that suggests anything negative. He says he has never thought of it in those terms, and he thinks most people plateau at that age. But he confirms that at the time he was having lots of fun, was unperturbed, genuinely at ease; there was nothing negative about that. Furthermore, his father had told him to try for a piece of the hog, not the whole hog, and he had had a good piece of the hog. Also, being realistic leads to tranquility and peacefulness. He didn't need to be greedy. And he certainly didn't need a big office staff or major political influence. Chet looks at me, senses my own struggles, and says with just a modicum of uncertainty, "Maybe I stopped running too early. But I did it consciously and without regret."

I know Chet intends no mockery of me. But we both know he has the advantage of having completed the age-fifty transition and can look back at it with the experience of a good 15 years. He knows, too, that after much soul-searching, I have recently resigned the leadership of a mental health center to accept yet another administrative promotion. He defined his plateau differently and at a point in time when I have opted for another spurt upward. He sets me thinking with his assertion that the most free people were nomads who worked only 2 hours a day to support their families. Then they played their music; recited their poetry; and used their time, space, and energy as they wished.

Chet concludes that he was pleased at age 55 with the idea of reaching his plateau. He exalts the notion of not having had to report to anyone and boasts of more individual freedom than the president of a university. We talk of the remarkable blessing of needing no more proof to feel accomplished and valued. The Harvard professorship conferred enormous respect and prestige. And he thought then, as he still thinks now, that few people could be luckier than he has been. So he stifles the idea that only emerges fleetingly and suggests he might have been hostage to his times and therefore settled for too little.

6

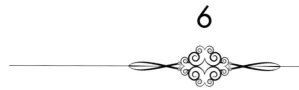

The Later Years

Chet Pierce suggests that my approach to talking about his life after 1982, my way of cutting his longitudinal development into segments, is somewhat forced because much of his life is repetitive after the 1970s. In making this point, he refers to his own developmental cycle by invoking once again the image of the plateau, reinforcing its steadiness and its lack of surprises and making it clear that it is a linear metaphor of stability and contentment. Chet obviously likes that thematic symbol, which makes me continually marvel at the general happiness that so characterizes his view of life. There is, at every turn, emphasis on how lucky he has been, his good fortune at having had the chance to do so much with his life, to have experienced so much love, to have seen so many different things, to have felt passion in a variety of forms.

I will not deny that the exercise of interacting with Chet forces me to consider whether I would evaluate my life in such positive terms. I know I engage in the assessment with more heaviness of heart and greater ambivalence than I have ever felt from Chet, who habitually blurts out his final conclusions with fluency and effusiveness and in vibrant language. I resort to subterfuges; I engage in pointless comparisons with other acquaintances; and I hear my parents' insistence that it is a slap against God to come out with anything less than an enthusiastic appreciation of the cards that life has dealt me. "Thank God for your mercies," they would urge. I even sense my embarrassment at being so pensive over my self-evaluation. Perhaps acquisition of the fluently positive vocabulary comes with the age-seventy transition, an obvious disadvantage for me, given where I presently stand on the timeline. Chet's words, coupled with the religion-based parental counsel, ring in my ears with a modicum of chastisement that I know he didn't mean for me. But I still hear his understated conclusion that he is very blessed. He had the capacity to have fun with opportunity and to pursue chances whenever he encountered them. He recognizes he had a better life than his father and even a better life than his children are likely to have, all because of his very good fortune.

I jump on his own use of language and ask once again why he was content with so little money. This time he is abruptly succinct. "I'm above it. Engaging in such negotiations is demeaning."

I ask, "Why is it demeaning to talk money?"

He replies, "I can't answer that."

He just reemphasizes the importance to him of controlling factors in his life such as time and space and adds that he is content to live in "relative genteel poverty." As another way of buttressing his position, he points out that Patsy is living in socioeconomic conditions that are superior to those in which she grew up. In contrast, he is living in relatively less impressive conditions than those that marked his early years, particularly during the Depression, when his father managed to provide well for the family. So if anyone has lost as a result of his choice, it is he.

As another way of conceptualizing the longitudinal evolution of his own timeline, I ask, even at the risk of being somewhat repetitive, that he think retrospectively about what he would say constitutes the major joys and disappointments of his life. We start first with his having completed his obligations as a father. He wanted to make sure his two daughters got an education that would prepare them for independent living, and he felt obliged to underwrite the cost. He is pleased that in return they were both ambitious and hardworking. He expands on his decision to send his younger daughter, Deirdre, on a trip around the world and explains how he tutored her for several months in an effort to prepare her thoroughly for the adventure. He alerted his friends at every stop so that she would always have support wherever she went, especially in the event of a health emergency. This is not the first time he has talked about this trip, and I grasp more clearly that he probably sees it as a special event in her life, marking some sort of turnabout. She's still not sure what she wants to do professionally, which leaves a certain number of question marks that I presume put the father side of Chet a bit off balance. He evidently worries for her, which is different from and more than just worrying about her. He senses her job is stressful and he would like so much to take everything on his own chin that is meant to hurt her even a little. Chet loves her generosity and regrets only that she does not have the vocational freedom and independence that he has enjoyed for so many years. He hopes he has supported her enough. Chet sees Deirdre as unusually thoughtful, kind, sensitive, and nurturing. He says that people comment often on the form and creativity she brings to interpersonal interactions.

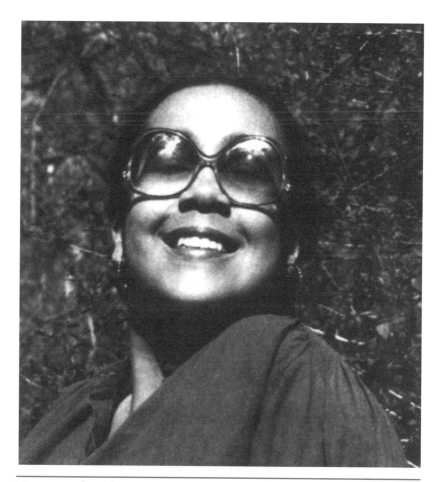

Younger daughter, Deirdre, circa 1995.

Chet's love for his children, and his contentment at seeing them reach maturity, is expressed in the language of protectiveness. His older daughter, Diane, now has three children, and Chet is concerned about the prolonged time her mothering tasks will take, especially because the responsibility of raising children always impacts on one's capacity to work and to develop seniority and expertise. He admires the strength needed to fulfill the mothering functions but is ambivalent about what being the wonderful mother does to the life of the professional woman. He hopes his grandchildren will have good opportunities in life, and he utters the minimalist type of regret I have come to associate with Chet. He is sorry that his two daughters will have more complicated lives than his has been, and he concedes he is disappointed that he will not be able to give financially as much to his children as he received from his own parents. I remain quiet, not making the point that I have previously argued more aggressively. But is this not clear proof of my position and the one that Samuel articulated so well? Money is not the major guarantor of happiness in life, but it serves certain functions and certainly can be employed judiciously to facilitate the achievement of particular objectives. Because of the generational difference, I have no doubt that Diane's husband, John Williams, understands my point. And I feel confident that Chet's grandchildren (Miguel, Ashley, and Arianna) will understand it even better. But that aside, Chet thinks about his grandchildren with profound love and concern. Once he even canceled an appointment with me because Miguel had called him up and invited himself to his grandparents' home. Even Chet loses control of his time when his grandchild calls.

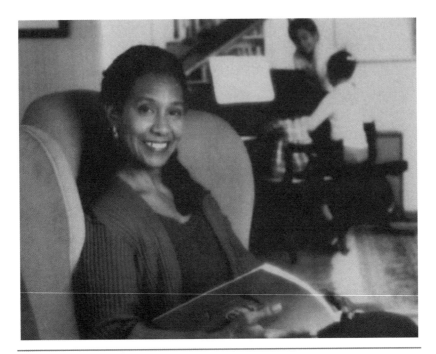

Older daughter, Diane, 1997.

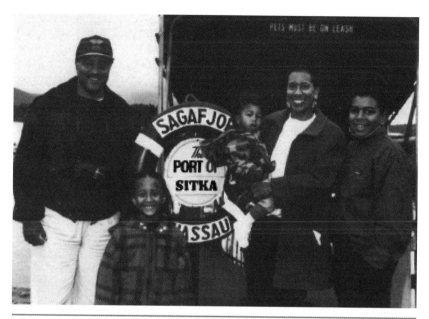

Diane Pierce Williams and family *(left to right)*: husband, John; daughters Ashley and Arianna; Diane; and son, Miguel.

Chet makes no automatic connection to Patsy's life, and I let that go temporarily. But I know from previous conversations it must be for her one of the major themes in her life with Chet, having given up so much to be the constantly supportive wife as well as the mother of his children. And she and Chet gave birth to only two. I shudder at the remembrance of my parents' bringing six children into the world of colonial Barbados, knowing well that my mother always maintained that she only carried out God's will. In her view, she had no choice, no encumbrances with decisions forced by the possibility of using birth control. Giving birth was giving life, and it was the lot of women. When I reflect on the way Chet talks, I realize that peeping through his words is the love of his independence and his marvelous experience of having had options from which to choose. I know from my brief encounters with Patsy that she will remain loyal to his decisions and his choices. Still, my mother's image haunts me, because I learned so late that she, too, was loyal and silent. The choices of the husband, despite what the familial conspiracy claims, are not necessarily the choices of the wife and mother. It is a lesson the men of my generation aren't rushing to digest too quickly. We know why. Giving the wife the same options we have strains the relationship and taxes all the professed claims of being patient and a believer in eq-

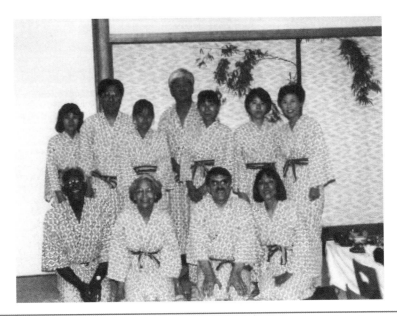

Chester and Jocelyn Pierce *(front row, left)* **with friends, circa 1993.**

uity and fairness. In short, being committed to the wife's equal access to opportunities demands energetic effort from the man.

So I sense some relief in Chet's voice when he says he is pleased that in the late 1970s Patsy decided to return to the university as a student, a point we discussed earlier, but one worth repeating. Apparently, the idea came up in a conversation between Patsy and someone who worked at the Boston University School of Social Work. Scholarship money was available, and there was some interest in older students. So Patsy took the plunge and enrolled in the master's degree program. Chet recounts a vignette that puts Patsy's decision into profound perspective and underlines my view of the concentrated commitment that must accompany talk of being interested in equality of opportunity for women. Before starting school again, she asked for help with the housework. Chet laughs, with unusual embarrassment, as he recalls how he asked her if she meant that she wanted him to do her work. He needs no nudging at all to appreciate how provocatively problematic his comment was, and in his own defense he can only mutter that he was, at the time, honestly seeking clarification of what Patsy was asking. I remember that at an earlier point in our conversations he had mentioned that it was likely Patsy would suggest he was more solicitous of their children's welfare than of hers. Of course, it is a commonly uttered indictment of husbands by their wives, and Chet sees it as a mere flicker on the broader screen of his relationship with Patsy.

After she finished the master's degree in social work, Patsy returned to full-time work, although in more recent years she has been working only 3 days a week as a coordinator of volunteer services. This reduced schedule has made it easier for her to accompany Chet on some of his travels, something she rarely did when taking care of the children was a central priority. Actually, travel together has always been a significant symbol in their collective lives, particularly travel by train. It has often meant something beautiful and positive, as in their first trip together when he took her to his home to present her to Hettie. Over the years, travel has also meant the freedom of Chet on the one hand and the restrictions of Patsy on the other hand. That is why, as Chet tells it, Patsy asked him not to come home talking about all the wonderful things he had just seen on his most recent journey. I can understand why Chet would relate his travel adventures to his family with passionate innocence. I can appreciate, too, why Patsy would hear his tales differently. After all, what symbolized his freedom characterized her lack of it. Travel certainly means something to Chet, as we know from the way it figures so prominently in his work and in his elaborately imaginative play with Uncle Ishkie, the shell fairy.

Nevertheless, when all is said and done, Chet sees Patsy as representing enormously good fortune in his life, and he is humbly apologetic that she and the family probably led a more routinized life over the years than his hectic, changing schedule permitted him. He also talks sensitively and somewhat haltingly, trying hard to cover up the pain, about her need to adapt to health problems, even though she has always appeared in the best of health. As she grows older, she is clearly more vulnerable, which is hard for the introspective Chet to take.

One of Chet's impressive areas of contentment has been the general domain of work. For one thing, he is pleased at having lived long enough to see a number of his students take jobs in the military, academia, and other contexts and to become successful. Some of them have been well placed to reciprocate kindnesses he had shown them at an earlier time, and they have invited him to participate in a well-paid consultation or to give a lecture. The success of his students justifies his existence as a teacher and makes it easier for him to think pleasantly of retiring.

The lecturing and the traveling often came together and provided Chet substantial satisfaction. He has given speeches at more than a hundred colleges and universities in the United States. I am struck by his pointing out that he has lectured on seven continents and worked as a psychiatrist in dozens of countries. He provides names of places I can only dream about—Siberia, New Zealand, Israel, Greenland, Yugoslavia, Fiji, Bolivia, Malaysia, Japan, the Philippines. He feels lucky to have traveled so much, and he likes the idea that the trips were distinctive if not distinguished. He is proud of the broad view of the world he has been afforded.

The special pleasure enjoyed in the professional arena has encompassed Chet's involvement with the National Aeronautics and Space Administration (NASA). In 1962, while working for Jay Shurley, Chet participated in the testing of female astronaut candidates. In 1966, he lectured in Houston on the comparison of space and Antarctica. After that, he was invited to talk at different meetings about a number of problems one could expect to arise in space travel, based on experience with other extreme environments such as the polar regions. So Chet held forth on such topics as the potential digestive problems of astronauts and problems female astronauts were likely to encounter in space. Later on, he was involved with the Soviets in work on psychological issues in space; he also chaired an international committee sponsored by the National Science Foundation and NASA to examine the applicability of polar region research findings to space. This led to further involvement with the NASA program, such as his membership on the task force to look at the bioethics of NASA initiatives. Chet is currently a member of the task force to advise NASA on the use of animals in space, and he is proud that his involvement with NASA has lasted for 30 years.

I bring to mind some conversations I have heard over the years in a number of different contexts with individuals explaining satisfaction with their work. I think especially of pastors, who have a way of articulating their specialness by making clear their proximity to God, or they derive pleasure from establishing an inability to escape the call from God, another way of justifying their supposed helplessness when God commands. Chet starts at another point entirely. He extols the luck and joy of being a physician, arguing that just by being a doctor, "people respond in confirming your sense of self, of worth." He also adds, "I never felt like I worked." And he always felt joyful about doing things, making a contribution, while remaining doubtful that many people intrinsically like their work. He brags, "What greater honor is there than having people share their greatest intimacies with you as a physician? Nothing beats being wanted. And a physician has a special privilege of not only feeling wanted, but also needed." A by-product of all this for Chet is that experiencing certainty about being affirmed has helped him believe in God and in the notion that he has been personally blessed. He won't go so far as to claim some special designation, but he knows benediction when he sees it, and he's confident of having had a lot of it. Furthermore, he's never had to seek out the affirmation; people just responded to him and made their positive comments and connections.

Chet returns to a point he had made earlier about the unique opportunity of a physician to do good in a concentrated fashion, in a way that in turn reinforces the physician's sense of self-worth. Chet emphasizes the point by turning to the Jim Jones story, an oblique reference that takes me a few minutes to straighten out. Jim Jones was, of course, the pastor who led his church flock to Guyana and supervised them as they all took poison and died. Sometime after that unfortunate event, Chet took part in a group assembled in San Francisco by the Fanon Center of Los Angeles to examine what led to the group suicide. During that time, they interviewed a survivor who gave a moving talk and explained that he was not among the dead because he had been away from the camp having his teeth fixed when Jim Jones announced the end. The interviewers asked the man how people could possibly have followed Jones. The reply was that Jim Jones let him do good whenever he wanted to, in sharp contrast to the larger community's restraint on doers of good works, in addition to the hesitancy in recognizing those who intend positive contributions to the society. Chet emphasizes that there are often restrictions on one's inclination to do good in addition to a corresponding lack of recompense. He wraps up the tangent by returning to his earlier assertion that doctors, even more than pastors, have a special opportunity to do good and to be esteemed by the society for their acts. It is at the very root of Chet's contentment with his profession.

Following the Watts riots in Los Angeles, Chet had served as a consultant in the establishment of the Drew Medical School and the Martin Luther King, Jr. Community Hospital. Located within the hospital was the Frantz Fanon Center, a Black mental health research facility. The Fanon entity was a byproduct of the Black Psychiatrists of America's lobbying of the National Institute of Mental Health.

Chet is pleased that he has always felt the obligation to do things in the wider community, and he links it to lessons from his parents. As a Black man, he has committed himself to a double obligation: to be a positive influence in the community and to work for the betterment of the Black community. At the same time, he was aware of his limitations when performing community service. For example, he didn't have the technique of raising funds, and he also felt the lack of administrative expertise. So he often managed to commingle the support he wished to give a community group with his professional interests, and he responded, for example, by conducting research for the organization. This approach did not work in every case, however, and Chet concedes his oc-

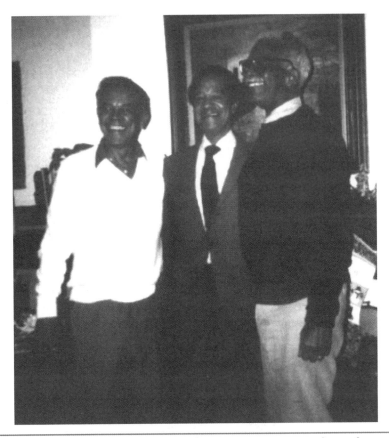

The Pierce brothers *(left to right)*: **Burton, Samuel, and Chester, 1996.**

casional disappointment when it was obvious the organization's board was not pleased by his inability to donate or recruit large sums of money.

In as disparaging a tone as I have ever heard from him, Chet makes it clear that his idea of a doctor's involvement in community service does not include being commodore of one's yacht club, something he had seen listed by a psychiatrist seeking to be elevated in a learned society. Doctors should be committed, through service, to helping the disadvantaged in the community, and Chet notes how persistent and ardent leadership of organizations can have an impact. He cites the influence of the Children's Television Workshop on television in general, largely through the dedication and leadership of its founders.

Chet moves on to cite the unusual experience and enormous pleasure of having known so many people from so many different walks of life, classifying these chances as perks that contributed to his having had a "more interesting life." For example, he has been in the dressing rooms at National Basketball Association and National Football League games. He has had the chance to know racketeers and movie stars; Nobel, Oscar, Emmy, Grammy, and Pulitzer Prize winners; celebrated musicians; and the presidents of Fortune 500 companies. He's been taken to dine at a U.S. senator's favorite restaurant, and he has had a tour of Los Angeles in one of that city's police helicopters. He's been given keys to major cities. A king has invited Chet to visit his country, and Chet has known prime ministers of other countries. These experiences have been informative and enriching and have provided him access to considerable influence, overriding any ephemeral attraction he might have had to money.

Riding this crest of Chet's personal contentment and appreciating the depth of my own vicarious pleasure, I ask him about Pierce Peak, a mountain located close to the South Pole, that was named after him in the mid-sixties. The explanation is amusing and simple. For years, Chet has been a member of the Antarctican Society, whose leader was an expert mapmaker. He was also the U.S. delegate assigned to the international group involved in naming places. As it turned out, if this man liked you, he would put your name on something, and not surprisingly, most members of the Antarctican Society have places named after them. Chet didn't ask for the honor; it just came in the mail. Chet also assures me there are thousands of peaks in the area to be named, so his Pierce Peak is no special achievement. Still, he has it listed in his curriculum vitae and he admits he is pleased by it. He laughs when I say, referring to his humility, that I've got him. And I laugh even more when he mounts an unconvincing defense and reminds me that Cicero noted that the person who wrote the treatise on anonymity signed his name. He closes the paragraph by poking more fun at me and stating that his daughters and he all have a very big map that is nicely framed and shows the location of Pierce Peak.

With such amusement at his own expense, we talk about his other honors. He has received two honorary Doctor of Science degrees, one from Westfield State College and the other from Tufts University. He can't recall what either of the citations said, and he has no knowledge of the factors that led to his selection. In May 1997, he was honored by the Wentworth Institute of Technology for "a lifetime of service in psychiatry, science, and education" and was given their degree of Doctor of Engineering Technology, *honoris causa*. But in general, he takes pleasure in the fact that his contributions have been recognized and that from time to time others have seen fit to make some public testimony about Chester Pierce and his work. He has been elected to the American Academy of Arts and Sciences. Colleagues nominated him for honorary membership in the Royal Australian and New Zealand College of Psychiatrists and in the Royal College of Psychiatrists in the United Kingdom. He has won awards from the American Psychiatric Association, the Black Psychiatrists of America, and the World Psychiatric Association. In 1971, one year after it was established, Chet was selected for membership in the Institute of Medicine at the National Academy of Sciences. Given that there are only 55 individuals in the Institute's Section of Psychiatry and Neurology, it is obvious that it is a signal honor. But Chet guards a particular sentiment for the decision of the National Medical Association to establish a special research seminar in his name, and he confesses to being substantively flattered by it, especially by the avowed objective of the seminar to attract Blacks to the research endeavor.

At another meeting, we return to the subject of Chet's joys and delights. He tells me that David Halberstam is writing a book about eight founders of one of the civil rights organizations and that two of the individuals had mentioned that Chet was a crucial force in their lives, evoking much appreciation from him. He observes that he has been asked to be a godfather, that books have been dedicated to him and children have been named after him, and that he's been asked to speak at weddings and funerals. And he has written testimonial letters on behalf of just about all the Black professors in his field. It has all been a pleasure. Chet is also struck by the length of uninterrupted time he has been a teacher. He is proud of the role he played in the National Medical Fellowships, a mechanism for distributing money to needy medical students. He won national and international awards for a short film he produced, and he is pleased that many people helped him in that project just at his simple request.

He then turns to an area of work that he was proud of, suggesting that he and I had not discussed it enough. He had a significant interest in capital punishment and had worked with Jolyon West and others to prepare an amicus brief for the U.S. Supreme Court when the Court was considering the constitutionality of capital punishment. Chet was against such extreme punishment and also argued that doctors ought not be involved in executions. As an informed forensic psychiatrist myself, I am weary of capital punishment discussions, and I leave the topic alone. It is the only subject I have not pushed Chet to elaborate on, and I wonder why. It is curious because Barbados remains among the few countries where hanging is still a possible punishment. In that island, where religion is a part of their cultural bedrock, hanging is still seen as a legitimate conclusion, particularly for those individuals who kill others with extreme viciousness.

I think Chet has spoken rather lucidly about his joys, and I dare to ask him what he would list as his major disappointments. At the top of the list is his regret that his children may not have as much joy and happiness in life as he himself has had. Then follows his concern about the future of his offspring, his nagging worry about whether he has supported them enough and whether their future is really assured. He turns then to talk about whether it would have been preferable for him to have concentrated his work in a particular area and to have become more of a specialist. Would his contributions have been more durable, then, if he had pursued some question in depth? Did he, in his own words, bet on the right horse?

He regrets not having followed through to develop a national forensic protocol. Because he thinks Blacks are likely to be incarcerated in increasing numbers, he believes that pressure should be brought to bear on the legal system so that it will be as fair as possible and that all inequities should be corrected. Chet insists that most judges would act differently if, as a group, they understood how they sentence Blacks to harsher jail penalties than Whites. So he underlines the need to highlight the sentencing data repeatedly. Chet is also sorry that he did not obtain money to organize a meeting of Black psychiatrists from throughout the diaspora. He apparently tried hard for 2 years and then gave up. He and I discussed that dream on several occasions, and I recognize it as part of Chet's wish to build solidarity among Black professionals. Chet instinctively knows the power of Black collectivity, and I have always powerfully agreed with him here.

It reminds me of a project I initiated a couple of years ago when I invited a group of Black and Hispanic pastors to work collectively on the task of considering the role that their churches could play in reducing the violence among New Haven's inner-city youth. Several pastors told me that this was the first time clergy from both ethnic groups had come together to work on an idea. The group successfully completed the specific agenda I had set for them. But it was also my broader hope that they would recognize the power and influence in their collective interaction. With the narrow task completed, they let their individual interests dictate the course of no longer meeting. I was disappointed but saw it coming long before it actually happened. I clearly understand Chet's regret.

Chet voices other regrets that I think are concordant with the task of looking back and taking stock. He is sorry that he's let drop contacts with certain people and places, especially because the people may not appreciate the tender place they occupy in his mind. He offers the example of Botswana, a place he has never seen but where he is confident there are a few people living who would have loved him. Chet regrets not having extended himself in all the many endeavors in which he was involved. Perhaps he did not do the very best job he could have done at the time. He recalls giving a paper at a conference, and someone asked him to stay in touch, but he didn't pursue it. The person turned out to be an individual who was in the process of forming a group that ultimately went on to write a seminal book about a futuristic society. Chet feels it an opportunity *manqué*, a peculiar reaction from someone who appears to have had so much. But he additionally reminds me that he has written about futurist matters and has presented papers at meetings of the World Future Society.

In contrast, his next two regrets evoke much more of my sympathy. First, he admits to never having resolved his feelings about leaving the Navy. He was about to go to the War College when he resigned his reserve commission, and Chet is confident that he was on the military's fast track. He stopped his involvement with the Navy at the rank of commander. I know how many times colleagues and I have engaged in second-guessing our career decisions. I realize this choice had extra urgency for Chet because I remember his stating that Patsy had enjoyed the lifestyle of a military wife. His other regret centered on his decision to give less time to playing the recorder and other musical instruments. He now thinks that decision might have been avoided had he organized his time better. Most people don't know of my own passion for congas and timbales or that I played those percussion instruments for years, finally letting them fall by the wayside when the professional time demands began to make leisure time interests too obvious a luxury. Of course, as we all get older, we recognize the folly of our distorted decision-making. But it's then too late to make up the lost time.

In talking about joys and disappointments, I turn the conversation to the only significant health problem I have ever heard Chet mention, which concerned his prostate. I hadn't understood that as far back as the late 1970s, while he was traveling in Australia, Chet had noted blood in his urine. On his return home, he consulted his urologist, the requisite laboratory studies were done, and the matter resolved itself. Around 1981, when he was once again in Australia, he found that he couldn't urinate. He had to be hospitalized and quickly catheterized. After he left the hospital, the problem recurred, which then required that the catheter be left in until his return to the United States. The prostatic hypertrophy was benign, and he ultimately underwent transabdominal resection, a technique that was recommended by the surgeons who saw him in Australia and back home. He took off the academic fall term that year, had the surgery, and recuperated leisurely. His only regret that year was having to turn down a visit to Malaysia when invited by the king.

Chet talks about the first time he confronted death squarely. He feels he faced, with substantial equanimity, the possibility of dying at the time he was awaiting the results of a biopsy that turned out to be negative. But he adds that one of his daughters thought he was not energetic enough in asserting a will to live. She disliked what she thought was his passivity. He disagrees with her view of it and says he was not looking forward to dying, although he was settled about the possibility. As he explains it, being settled did not mean he wasn't going to do his best to stay alive. He believes that perhaps the only test of maturity is how one faces death. He adds that in light of what God has given him, he has no right to regret leaving this world.

I ask how he had discussed the prostate surgery with Patsy. His reply is that they talked about it with the same flavor. He made sure she knew where certain important things, such as the will, were located in the house. But there was really nothing that either of them could do to make a difference in the outcome of the problem. He also argues that he was well prepared for the experience through his interactions with patients and that he knew the possible extreme consequences. He recalls how disabling the symptoms were, including the urgency to urinate as well as the lack of control over the urinary mechanism. Chet waxes philosophical about the need to cope with one's declining capacities, insisting that as time marches on, we all have to be more modest in our expectations. We instinctively follow the tangent to another road not talked about much in public, but one we both know so well as physicians, because God in his master plan linked urination to other functions. And Chet says, comically, that when it was hard, it was very, very hard. But when it was soft, it was very, very soft—and that was bad. "One has to cope with memories and be thankful. The thing is to know that 200 years ago, if I had prostate trouble, I would be dead."

He and I had not talked much about death, and I ask him if he knows how his life is going to end. There is, of course, no artful posing in the question. It is no more than an unsophisticated technique to broach a topic that makes us all uncomfortable. Chet ignores the gauche approach and replies that it would be a great boon to die happy. He says he can think of diseases and deaths he wouldn't like to have, such as one caused by pemphigus, the severe skin disease. So he will continue to hope for a happy end. The discussion reminds him of being called to Dr. Ralph Bunche's deathbed to say adieu to him. Chet was at Meharry when a telephone call came that summoned him to Bunche's bedside. By the time he arrived, Bunche was no longer talking. But Chet recalls their squeezing each other's hand, and he is confident the cellular connections allowed him to transmit his thanks to Bunche, who had, with no provocation, gone out of his way to help Chet on several occasions. The experience with Bunche was truly powerful, and it has taught Chet about being humble in the face of death. "Until you face death, you don't know how mature you are." It is a natural step at this point to talk about God once more. Chet reaffirms his belief in God, but he admits his uncertainty about everlasting eternity. Like most of us, he hopes that if the Kingdom really exists, he'll make it through the pearly gates. He would like a reunion with his parents and his descendants, although he cannot tell how much is hope and how much is belief. So he's not sure about the existence of an afterlife, just as he's not sure about the divinity of Jesus. He caps his thinking in this arena with the uncomfortable avowal, "I'm too puny in my thinking to get through a lot of things." I do not dwell on it, because it is the admission of a brilliant mind conceding that he cannot box with God or with the force that runs things from up there or out there. I prefer his humility in throwing in the towel in these discussions.

It takes me back to innumerable discussions on the topic of death with my pastor-father, who in his own right was a first-class preacher. I always told him the only really bad sermon I ever heard him preach was at funerals, when he'd stand there trying to explain why some 10-year-old innocent child had just been mowed down by some idiot's bullet. My father would invent all kinds of pointless explanations for the gratuitous loss of life, and I would turn fretfully in my seat because I couldn't believe anyone in the church really bought the illogic of his reasoning. And I was embarrassed for him. Why could he not reduce the pain and just say his mind was too limited to spar with God on these matters of death? Actually, I do remember one occasion when he did preach a first-class funeral sermon. He had changed his technique by then. He told the congregation the deceased was in God's hands; then he turned to asking about the salvation of those who were in the church, alive and still in possession of the luxury of being able to contemplate death. I liked that.

Discussing death and dying sooner or later takes its toll, and I preferentially move to a counterfeit symbol, Chet's retirement. It is fortuitous that Chet and I had a meeting on March 1, 1996. After a previous session when we talked so much of the potential loss of the one individual who has so clearly been his life partner, he greeted me with the decision that he had decided to retire. This interrupted the natural flow of his story and of our dialogue, but the issue was on his mind, and he would not sit on it. March 4 was his birthday, and on that day, the ritual-conscious

Chester Pierce submitted—no, hand-carried—his resignation, to be effective July 1, 1997. I counted six people who received the letter on the same day and from Chet's own hand because it was "the gentlemanly thing to do." He judged that six letters were required because he had to inform all the different people with whom he was officially connected in the three different faculties and multiple departments or divisions.

I was astounded once again by the complexity of this man. He persistently asserted that he is not really a Harvard man, but even in retirement he behaved with class and style and respect for its institutions. I half stifled the unkind thought that certainly few of the recipients of the letter would even appreciate the significance of the ritual that Chet observed; and I certainly wondered whether they could think it more than mere accident, even if they grasped the import of the ritual. In the scheme of things, even at Harvard, I wondered who cared anymore, who had the time to reflect on the nature of what constitutes a gentleman, a Black one at that. But Chet was in a reflective mood, and he noted that it would really be "withering" for institutions like Harvard if all the professors stayed on past age 70. He let me in on some of his other fears that day, especially regarding his contemplated retirement.

Chet notes he has already started to reduce the amount of traveling he usually does and he is less inclined to participate in all the social activities that generally are expected of him. He is also becoming more sensitive to what everything costs, and he is constrained to acknowledge that his buying power has actually decreased over the years, which means he is relatively poorer than he was a few years ago. Because we are talking about money, I ask him about his usual fashion of negotiating his salary, and he simply shocks me by saying that he has never negotiated a salary. He has always just accepted what he was offered. At the same time, he makes it clear he has never made a move because of money. The decision to move to Oklahoma had nothing to do with salary. He puzzles me more by explaining that he has always recognized the likelihood that he would earn less and probably have to do more than his White colleagues. But using his own personal logic, he is pleased that his style of doing things has kept him less beholden to his employers. I am also struck by his added comment that he has never had a set fee for any of his lectures and has simply just accepted what he was offered. Such heroics are dimmed a bit by the reality of retirement, and Chet is concerned that the cessation of paid employment will cause the diminishing of what little he has to leave his children.

Naturally, I wonder about the connection of salary and lecture fees to one's self-esteem. Chet resists my logic. He counters with the notion that he has always felt fairly compensated, and in accepting the salary offered, he has then always turned and defined a number of activities that he excluded from his portfolio. For example, he did not attend faculty meetings and would not serve on committees that he considered of no real value. In Oklahoma, he eschewed the committees but would then spend considerable time in community projects, such as work with the police leadership.

I can't help commenting about some of my colleagues who I know have turned salary negotiation into a fine art, and we start down the tangent talking about some of these same colleagues who love as much publicity as they can get. I probably make the connection that these colleagues think publicity enhances their worth at salary negotiation time. Chet responds without blinking an eye, and we discuss our professional colleagues freely. Chet has rarely sought publicity, and he thinks it usually makes no sense for Blacks to be in the media at a frequency that is way out of proportion to their actual representation in the society. At the same time, he points out that he has always taken seriously the task of developing deep relationships with key people in any community. But to Chet, being critically influential has nothing to do with one's visibility. I note that Chet opted to have access to influence and power through the quiet pursuit of excellence, and I ask him what he thinks of my own obvious technique that I learned well from other mentors whom he in fact knows. I mention the administrative style of having control over resources. Chet laughs with facile recognition in his eyes and reminds me that he turned down the offer to be associate dean at the Harvard Medical School and has pursued no departmental chairmanships. I also think he humors me a bit by conceding that personality makeup dictates or strongly influences our preferences in this kind of choice. But I retort that some managers like myself also prefer to manage resources quietly and with minimum fuss. It's clear we agree that our love of anonymity dictates much of what we do, although we both also recognize that telling stories publicly can't possibly be the surest way to keep secrets.

Chet thinks this business of being critically influential is related to the art of deciding where you allocate your energy. He would join an important committee to accomplish a clearly defined task he thought important, but once the defined work was over, he would move on to other things, always resolutely controlling his time and energy. That is always for Chet a major issue—that Blacks should work hard at controlling their time so as to be able to allocate it judiciously to specific tasks, with the ultimate desired effect of enhancing their effectiveness. Chet agrees that temperament and chance also influence how each person makes the decision. But he goes on to make one more point, that for

Black professionals it is a mistake to keep only a Black portfolio. He argues that if Blacks are always funneled into pursuing Black causes and questions, it makes it easy for Whites to dismiss us. In his view, Blacks must learn to take on issues with cosmopolitan applicability. This is a way of answering my critics who felt I should never have moved to Yale.

All the studied reflection almost makes me forget it was Chet's contemplated retirement that served as the catalyst, and I realize now that I've been encountering this theme in protean forms—references to a limited number of supervision hours yet to complete, comments about rejected invitations to lecture because they require too much travel or preparation, and so on. His impending retirement naturally reminds me that during this age-fifty transitional period, I have been considering altering my own work plans. The thoughts are hard to formulate logically and publicly. Still, I think them nothing heroic in comparison to reaching the conclusion that one will give up work. I wonder, too, if Black men think about retirement differently from White men, and I also wonder about Chet's view of this.

We return to the retirement, and Chet repeats that he feels honor in adhering to the ground rules that previously required his retirement at age 70. For him, there is grace in relinquishing his post now. He contends that the old professors must get out, otherwise the younger generation will be stifled. Besides, there will be no loss to the world if he leaves. Not to do so would be selfish. On the other hand, he rejects any idea of celebrating his departure. He thinks it would be dishonest to do so because he was never a social person. Besides, who would come, he asks, and he additionally dislikes the notion of self-promotion. Of course, we have certainly discussed this theme before. He adds more weight to his argument about never wanting to be unnecessarily in the limelight by showing me a letter he received recently inviting him to participate in a book on Harvard. The author wanted to write about Chet's having played in the 1947 football game against the University of Virginia. In effect, he was the first Black to play football against a White Southern school. But Chet thinks his contribution was minimal. The game may have been a historic occasion in the context of the 1940s, but Chet insists he just happened to be there.

I experience disappointment in his refusal to be saluted as he takes leave of a long and illustrious career at Harvard. There was, in fact, actual funding for the occasion. Tony Earls, a Black professor at Harvard and a mutual friend, and emeritus professor Leon Eisenberg had obtained about $10,000 from the three Harvard faculties and Massachusetts General Hospital to underwrite a farewell for Chet. So I launch a direct attack on his point of view. After all, my engagement in this exercise of studying his life positions me to make a speech of some sort at an event set up to celebrate him. I know his life fairly well by now, and I could be eloquent. Chet won't budge, however, and he raises the specter of "improbable people" attending some shindig in his honor. He illustrates the concept of improbable presence by talking about funeral ceremonies, where there is always a mourner present who has no conceivable connection to the deceased. However, the individual shows up at the ritual and often is very visible. Chet can foresee some improbable people participating in some ritual meant to honor him, and that gives him added strength to resist the idea. Furthermore, he knows the people who genuinely appreciate him, and he has no need to celebrate that in public. He then mentions his fear that he isn't well known at Harvard because he has always "existed quietly." I wonder how deep the insecurity is but will not pursue it.

Chet brings up the name of a Black emeritus Harvard professor, Harold Amos, whom I do not know. But Amos is a famous cancer researcher whose achievements Chet admires and who has had substantial impact on Harvard students, particularly with persuading Black science students to enter research careers. Chet makes the point that Amos has for many years played a crucial role at Harvard as a professor and former head of the Medical School's Department of Microbiology. Yet when Amos retired, Chet was unaware of his change in status. This is Chet's model: quiet excellence. Chet knows I like this model of reserved distinction, particularly because it suits my temperament. But I point out how I have learned well over the years that, especially in the political marketplace, theatrics and noise are sometimes useful. Chet does not disagree.

I bring up again his wish to dispense unilaterally with the ritual of marking the end of his tenure. He emphasizes his preference not to support the ritual. He does not like it or want it. And why put so much stock in one evening after all the years he has given to Harvard? He sees himself as just going off the payroll, and he does not expect his life to be much different after retirement. He hasn't even considered asking for an office, as emeriti faculty are often provided. But he assures me he will ask for a key to the building so he can use the bathroom facilities whenever he's walking around in Harvard Square and feels the need.

I give up the struggle, as I feel one must in these situations. After all, I must concede that Chet has the right and indeed the privilege of defining what the formal end of his career will look like. I would like to honor him, to give him the gift of some ritualized celebration. He can say he doesn't want it. He talks more sensibly of this important aspect of the age-seventy transition than I ever expect to do. I speak of the passage into a new status that is no longer so formidably defined and characterized by one's work and profession. I hope I will handle the change as gracefully as Chet does and will not be afraid to imitate him, as he speaks clearly of the fact that his career is now over. There is no project still to be done, he says. There are things to occupy him, but nothing driving him to be involved in the stream of the profession. There are no conferences he feels he must attend, no organization whose structure and function he must still influence. There is no special place he feels he has to go.

I take the final risk of asking Chet what he thinks now about having participated in the dialogue with me. He acknowledges some unexpected benefits and declares that the dialogue has been instructive. There are many questions he would never have posed to himself, and he expects the text will be a wonderful legacy for his descendants. But he states, too, that the introspection was not all pleasant or positive. He realizes he had good fortune, and many things took place in happy circumstances. But he also saw his shortcomings. He muses about whether he extended himself enough, whether he did the right thing with what he had and made the most of every opportunity. It is the closest he has come to formal therapy. I cringe a bit because it is not quite the word I would have used, although I recognize the significance of his statement. I suppose I wondered afterward whether he was implying that I had behaved like a therapist, a role I could never embrace in contemplating my approach to the task of producing narrative. He concedes I made him think about how passive he was in his life. From time to time, I also put more emphasis on certain topics than he would have done, and he grants that ultimately my truth is as good as his.

"In any society, a man who is 70 is an elder. You've had your time. And in my case, it has been a wonderful time. I know lots of guys who'd have liked to live as long as I have. It's been marvelous. As Casey Stengel said when he turned 70, 'Most people my age are already dead.'"

That is Chet's assessment of what his own life has meant to him. It is his view of it, his thoughts of what he has tried to do, or meant to do. I promised to hold his feet to the fire, to make the dialogue as sensible as I could, to contend with what I learned about a hero of mine. I know the journey for him has required considerable courage and stamina. But he stayed the course, and I learned a lot about the business of looking back thoughtfully at the ineffaceable footprints one has left behind.

Appendix

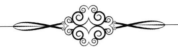

This section houses the birthday thoughts penned in 1982 by Chester Pierce and the children's stories that he wrote to his daughters when on travel away from home. These two examples of his unique writing style were placed elsewhere in the original edition. Also added here are typical examples of correspondence between him and the author. The letter written in poem form from Richard Fournier to Ezra Griffith celebrates and memorializes the 1998 publication of *Race and Excellence*. The final document is a testament to Professor Pierce after his passing in 2016. The 2017 memorial celebration commemorates his passing and records the names of family and friends who commented on his life. This appendix effectively presents other dimensions of his life as father, philosopher, friend, and humanist.

Birthday Thoughts: 1982

Then the short-lived genes course from the despairing heart to the restless mind, professing what they believe to be true: "This man has had the best that Fortune offers—a loving and tender woman."

The gods jest and sport so that only the good might master the game of life and only the fortunate can discover how it is scored. Perhaps points are scored only for serving, loving, and caring. Perhaps the game's goal is to balance matchless regrets against unforgettable boons.

My matchless regrets are these:

- Not to have been with people whom I know I would enjoy
- Not to have seen places I know I would have cherished
- Not to witness the autopsy I could most inform
- Not to absorb the past and future unhappiness of those I love
- Not to see how this world turns out in a hundred or a thousand years

Yet unforgettable boons overpower these towering and unyielding regrets. For I have had it said to me, "Stay with me...let me come...don't go now...come back soon." And I have said to myself, "I will die happy, for I have savored and gained the greatest boon that mortals can know."

The older I get the more value I place in the lesser as opposed to the greater virtues. The greater virtues are wisdom, justice, and intelligence. Lesser virtues are qualities such as gentleness, kindness, cheerfulness, joy, and gratefulness.... Now I am coming to the view that the lesser virtues in fact are ancestors and commanders to the greater virtues.

Chester Pierce, M.D.

Children's Tales

The Amazonian Dolphin

In the Amazon River in South America there live some ferocious little fish who have big, sharp teeth. The fish are called piranha. These little fish travel in teams of dozens, searching for food. Wherever piranha swim, people must be very careful. If any meat is placed in the water, the piranha, with their big, sharp teeth, will swarm to it and eat it all up in a matter of seconds. Naturally they are unpopular and feared, for anything so unfortunate as to be in the water with them is completely eaten up.

One day long ago, in an Indian village on the Amazon River, the favorite puppy of the village decided it was so hot that he'd take a swim. The puppy dog didn't know about the dangerous piranha. Before anyone saw him, the dog was swimming happily in the water.

The Indians ran to the shore and called for him to come back. But the puppy was too happy and he made believe he didn't hear them. No one could jump into the water to save him because everyone feared the fish. Some of the grownups ran to their canoes, but already the people on the shore saw the ripples on the water, indicating that the piranha, with their big, sharp teeth, were heading for the little dog. Everyone was very upset, because the dog was loved almost as much as any child or adult in the village. He could do all sorts of tricks and he was always friendly, happy, and fun to be around. Now it seemed he was to be eaten up by the terrible fish.

Just then a large fishlike animal jumped out of the water and headed for the puppy dog. Now everyone believed the piranha would have two meals: one of a dog and one of a fish. Yet, this big fishlike animal swam right into the piranha. Instead of being eaten up, he began to eat. The dozens of little piranha scattered. They swam as fast as they could in order to get away from this creature.

After driving off the fish, the large animal swam back to the puppy dog, who had paddled around in the water enjoying all the excitement. The large fishlike animal let the dog play for a little while and then gently prodded the puppy back to shore.

This big animal was an Amazonian dolphin. When the people on the shore recognized the dolphin as he brought in the puppy, their glee made them yell with delight. They were very thankful to get back their little dog. Besides, they were especially happy to know that there existed an animal who could chase away the hungry piranha.

Now it happened that these Indians loved to have parties with much feasting and dancing. The Indians decided to have a celebration that night because the terrible piranha had been beaten.

At the celebration, the chief of all the Indians said, "From now on, whenever we have a feast we'll leave a place of honor, at the head of our table, for our friend the dolphin." Someone else suggested that they make a very special hut and keep it as comfortable as possible, in the event that the dolphin ever visited them.

The girl who owned the puppy was the prettiest girl in the village. She suggested that at every celebration the prettiest girls should be available to dance with the dolphin, in the event that he ever visited them.

So it occurred that for years later in Amazon Indian villages, at each celebration, there was a place of honor set aside for the protector against the piranha. The strongest boys in the village made it their duty to keep a comfortable hut in readiness in case the dolphin ever visited. At the feast, the prettiest girls never entered the dances around the campfire. They waited in case the dolphin would come to visit.

In truth, no one really believed the dolphin would ever visit. They knew that it lived in water. Besides, they knew the dolphin wasn't aware that he was so honored by them. Finally, they used to say that the dolphin would be unhappy if he visited because he didn't speak their language.

Many more years passed by. The villagers continued to keep all their special honors for their friend and protector, the dolphin. Yet everyone in the village, from the youngest to the oldest, never really expected a visit from the dolphin.

What these good people didn't realize was that the dolphin did know he was honored and that he could live out of the water for a little while. And he talked their language. The dolphin decided to go to the very next feast.

When it was time for that celebration, all the people from a number of villages gathered together to enjoy themselves. Suddenly everyone stopped eating. The drums stopped beating. Even the noises in the jungle quickly stopped. For there in the midst of the gathering, near the campfire, stood a 7-foot dolphin.

This was surprise enough, just to see a great fishlike animal standing on his tail. But even more surprising was that he wore a red beret and dark eyeglasses. To everyone's further surprise, he swaggered over to his place of honor. Here the villagers were in for their greatest surprise. In a hushed voice, with a soft breathlessness, the dolphin said, "Hi guys, hello girls!"

After they got over their astonishment, the Indians were extremely happy. After all these years their protector had come to visit. The Indians presented every generosity they knew to their long-honored friend. They brought all sorts of fruit and meat for him to eat. But he seemed more interested in talking to the people. He asked them all about themselves. He told them all about life in the Amazon River.

Soon it was time for the dancing to begin. Imagine everyone's surprise when this gigantic dolphin stood up, bowed gracefully to the prettiest girl in the village and in a hushed voice, with a soft breathlessness, said, "I believe this dance is mine." Everyone was thrilled that the dolphin knew and appreciated all the honors he had been given for being their protector against the piranha. By now the evening had been so full of surprises that no one thought it amazing to see a dolphin dancing with all the girls. He talked to all the guys. Never had there been such a joyous occasion in all of South America.

Suddenly the dolphin announced it was time for him to go to bed. He assured the good villagers that he knew he had a special hut and he could find his own way to his lodgings.

One little girl tugged at his flipper and said she had a question to ask. The little girl's mother and father grew anxious, for their little girl sometimes asked embarrassing questions. They knew from the look on her face that she was about to ask the honored guest such a question.

Before she could be stopped, she said, "Dolphin, why do you wear a red beret and dark eyeglasses?" Once again everyone stopped eating. The drums stopped beating. The jungle stopped chattering. Naturally everyone wanted to know the answer, but no one had asked the question because they thought the dolphin might have his feelings hurt. However, to their great relief, the dolphin seemed unannoyed by the question. He looked down at the little girl and said in a hushed voice, with a soft breathlessness, "It's to give me some style and dash."

With that he bid the villagers goodnight and swaggered off to his hut. As he left, the strongest boy in all of the villages cried out, "I've never seen a dolphin with more style and dash!"

When the dolphin got to his hut he lay down. He was famished. He had danced and partied but had had no fish to replenish his strength. Therefore, he knew he couldn't stay out of the water much longer. Had he eaten he would have been able to remain at the party longer. He hadn't told his hosts that he ate only fish because a dolphin with so much style and dash was very careful to be always courteous to his hosts. He lay quietly on the palm leaf bed that had been made for him. After a while, he heard everyone leave the party and go home to bed.

The next morning the strongest boys woke up early and went to the jungle to find all the favorite fruits that boys love. These they brought back to the special hut. It was the strongest boys who discovered the dolphin had gone. They shouted their grief and the entire village woke up.

The village drummer beat the message to other villages. Soon the jungle was filled with drumbeats. The village chief arrived at the hut and saw for himself that indeed their guest had departed.

Everyone crowded around the hut. The villagers all cried because they missed their guest. Some looked forward to seeing his dark eyeglasses and red beret. Others said they would like to once again hear his hushed, breathlessly soft voice. All the guys wanted to talk to him. All of the girls wanted to dance with him. The children wished to imitate his style and dash as he swaggered about being polite and considerate to everyone he met.

The little girl who had asked the question was the first to notice some writing on a palm leaf (of course, by now no one was astonished that the dolphin could write). The chief picked up the palm leaf and muttered to himself that he had never seen penmanship that showed so much style and dash.

He read aloud the message from their protector. It said, "Dear Friends, Thank you all for the kindness you extended to me. Please excuse my abrupt departure, but I had to return to the river to get my breakfast. Always I will keep you in my thoughts. Never, ever will I forget your wonderful celebration. Whenever I can, I will come back to visit you."

Many people don't believe that a dolphin comes ashore ever so often to join a party. Yet, there are numerous villages in South America that keep ready an honored place for the dolphin. Their strongest boys keep a luxurious hut for him. Their prettiest girls all think that someday they will dance with a gallant, 7-foot dolphin, whose red beret and dark eyeglasses give him style and dash.

Recently, visitors to the Amazon River reported that men's lives had been saved when they fell into the water and were threatened by the fierce piranha. A large fishlike animal had arrived and scattered the little fish with the big, sharp teeth. Some visitors even have said that the dolphin, believe it or not, wears a red beret and dark eyeglasses.

One visitor hesitated, out of shame, to tell his story, for he didn't expect anyone to believe it. However, he says that once, while his boat was passing through waters known to be filled with piranha, he heard a great swirling in the water. All the passengers looked out and there they saw a dolphin with a red beret and dark eyeglasses. He waved his flipper at them, and in a hushed, breathlessly soft voice he said, "Hi guys, hello girls!" This visitor said he had never seen a dolphin with so much style and dash. But then, too, he knew no one would ever believe him. Do you?

I Am a Kiwi

I am a kiwi. I'm a bird. You won't believe it, but some of my closest relatives were the moas, the largest birds that ever inhabited the earth (in fact, next to the elephant and giraffe, they were taller than any living mammal). The rest of my family includes the emu, the cassowary, and the rhea. And of course, you know my cousin, who hides his head in the ground, the ostrich.

Why have you never seen me? Well, I come from a long, long way off. Even where I live, I only go out in the darkest part of night. Then I use my sense of touch and hearing to show me the way to the roots, insects, and worms that I live on. As a special treat, I eat any ripe fruit that happens to be on the ground. However, I'm very nervous, and as soon as I eat, I scurry back into my home in the bushes long before the light of day.

But you still don't believe I'm a bird. I know people always say that birds should fly. I can't fly anymore than you, for like you, I have no wings. It doesn't bother me that I can't fly — well, not too much—because after all, lots of birds can't fly. Like who? Like the penguin, for instance, who is one of the best swimmers alive—but still can't fly.

Since you seem to like me and seem to care about me, I'll tell you a secret which I've never told anyone. Right now I can't sing. I can whistle a high-pitched note that sounds as if I say the word "kiwi." That is how I got my name. But once upon a time I had a beautiful voice. Even relentless time would stand still while I sang. Well, if you don't believe that, you won't believe that once upon a time even before I had my beautiful voice, I was a beautiful woman. In fact, I was so beautiful that people said that only Orion, the handsomest man who ever lived, was suitable for me to marry.

As so often is the case, the great beauty brought me troubles. For one day as I sat admiring myself, I had an impious thought. I thought that my beauty made me more irresistible to men than the vaunted beauty Aphrodite. Aphrodite heard this thought, for it was she who gave me beauty. She used to like to reside in my mind so that she too could enjoy all the nice things that happen only to the extraordinarily beautiful. As a result of this impious thought, she said, "Irresistible you are. Henceforth, men will die for your beauty."

At that point she changed me into a Siren. As you know, a Siren is a bird who has the face of a beautiful woman. Sailors on the ocean hear the lovely bird's voice and are compelled to find it. As they get nearer, they see the face of a fabulous beauty and they become careless of their seamanship and crash their vessels. Such was my role as a Siren who seduced sailors to their deaths.

However, I was still proud. Oh, what an awful sin! Therefore I used to admire the music I made as a bird. Surely, I thought, this is just recompense for not being a woman. For no woman or goddess could make such beautiful music. In fact, in my loneliness I used to talk to the heavens, and one day I told this very thought to the stars.

The constellation Gemini heard it. The twins, Castor and Pollux, had a double grievance with me. In the first place, my music and looks were so charming that sailors had wrecked themselves even before they could beseech the Gemini, the guardians of storm-beset sailors. In the second place, they had not liked it when I was a woman and people said I was more beautiful than their sister, Helen. For she was so striking that a war was fought over her when she was a child. Again, when she was an adult, her beauty caused a thousand shiploads of men to leave Greece to besiege Troy for 10 dreadful years. Thus the twins were glad to hear my boast, and they told the Muses.

The Muses appeared and challenged me to a music contest. The loser was to be humiliated in whatever fashion the winner decided. The judges of the contest were the famous mythical minstrel, Orpheus, and the superb virtuoso, King Amphion. Many music lovers appeared at the contest, including Hermes, Athene, Aphrodite, and Apollo. I saw also Pan and Sileneus. Later, I was told that Midas and Marsyas were there, as were Herakles, Chiron, the Nymphs of the oceans and the Nymphs of the woods.

It was a hard-fought contest, and even today I dare not think how worthy an opponent I was, since I know impious and insolent thoughts have been my undoing. After 3 days and 3 nights of contesting (amidst the thunderous applause of the spectators), I was declared the loser—but a worthy one. All spectators agreed to the fairness of the verdict, particularly the indication that I was worthy. For this meant that there was recommendation for clemency.

My humiliation was to be the loss of my woman's face, my voice, and my bird's wings. My clemency was that I was exiled to the end of the world, where I would live forever in a country of unequaled beauty. And that is where you find me now, in beautiful New Zealand, where I venture out only at night. I fear that someone may see me and know that I was thinking to myself, "I once was more beautiful than Helen and I once almost won a contest from the Muses."

So please don't tell anyone my secret, for I may suffer more wrath from powerful ones. That's why I'm so nervous. Please keep me near you, in a dark place, like under your bed. And if you take me out and pet me every once in a while (in the dark, of course), I will tell no one that there is someone special in your life. This someone thinks that you too are as beautiful as Helen and as inspiring as a Muse. And do you know who that special person might be? Yes, it is your own Uncle Friendly Bear.

Oh yes, Uncle Friendly Bear the philologist (philologist means lover of words) has tried to find out what Kiwi means. It is the only word the Muses left me. Uncle Friendly Bear thinks there is no Greek origin for the word. However, he has good reason to know that it means, "I love you every time you pick me up to pet me." Kiwi! Kiwi!

The Grasshopper

Would you like to be an entomologist? An entomologist studies insects. But even an entomologist wonders about the first grasshopper. Every child of ancient Greece thought he knew because of the story of Eos and Tithonos.

Eos was the goddess of dawn. She fell in love with a man named Tithonos. Since Eos was a goddess, she was immortal and would never die.

Tithonos, being a man, was a mere mortal. He knew that it would be dangerous for him to love a goddess. But each day before dawn pushed back the night, Eos reached from her heavenly couch to touch Tithonos. She was so beautiful and tender that he could not resist returning her love. And so Eos and Tithonos became very much in love.

One day Eos went to Zeus with a special request.

"O, great ruler of the universe," she began. "My beloved Tithonos is a man. Since all men someday die, I am afraid I will lose him. Please, O wise and just Zeus, please allow Tithonos to live forever."

Selene, the moon goddess, was the sister of Eos. She too went to Zeus. "Great and powerful Zeus," she said, "my sister Eos is so unhappy. She worries that Tithonos might die. Please make this man immortal."

Eos also had a brother. His name was Helios. Helios was the god of the sun. "Radiant light of heaven," he pled, "have mercy on beautiful Eos. Return her happiness. Grant Tithonos life forever."

Zeus listened to Eos and Selene and Helios. He listened to many other gods and goddesses who came to add their pleas.

Finally he spoke, "Beautiful Eos, rosy-fingered goddess of the morn, my heart is softened by your sadness. I will grant your wish. But beware of the consequences when a mere mortal loves a goddess."

Eos was so happy that she ignored the warning of Zeus. She jumped on her wonder horse, the winged Pegasus, and hurried to tell Tithonos the wonderful news.

Remember that wise Pegasus could not only fly but could also talk. And as they soared across the heavens, he spoke. "Lovely Eos," he said, "it brings great joy to me when you are happy. I know that you received everlasting life for Tithonos, but tell me, did you also receive everlasting youth for him?"

The happiness of Eos turned to grief. "Oh, Pegasus," she moaned, "I forgot. I asked just for the immortality of Tithonos. I forgot to ask that he stay young forever, as gods and goddesses do."

In spite of the grief of Eos, she and Tithonos knew much happiness. Perhaps their greatest joy was the son born to them. He was a beautiful Ethiopian named Memnon.

As time went by, Tithonos did in fact become old and feeble. Eos, of course, remained young and full of energy. When Tithonos was no longer able to use his arms and legs, yet still could not die, Eos suffered quite as much as he did. Finally the gods could no longer bear his suffering and turned him into a grasshopper.

Memnon, the beautiful son of Eos and Tithonos, became king of the Ethiopians. He fought bravely and died a hero during the Trojan War.

Eos, seeing her son's fate, returned Memnon to Africa. There, in the land of the pyramids, stood two gigantic pillars. One was called Memnon's. And it was said that when the first rays of morning fell upon this statue, a sound like the plucking of a harp string could be heard. This sound was believed to be Eos mourning for her son. Perhaps this is the sound made when the heart of a goddess breaks. The early morning dewdrops were thought to be her tears.

And each morning at dawn, there was also a grasshopper who joined the woeful wailing.

Do you think an entomologist could tell you how sad a grasshopper can be?

The Girl Who Lost Her Shadow

She made everyone happy and gay. That's why she was called Joy. When she smiled, everyone smiled. And when she laughed, even the sunshine felt warmer. Best of all, Joy was always kind to other people. In short, everyone who looked on her was in love with her. And everything she looked upon, she loved.

One day Joy took some friends down to the seashore. One of them accidentally got water in her mouth and said, "Ooooh, that tastes *awful!*"

Another friend decided to take a swim, but when she stepped into the water, she screamed and ran back. "The water is *terrible!*" she cried. "It's so *cold!*"

Joy's third guest just sat and looked at the water. "I wouldn't go *near* the ocean," she said, "it's so big, I'm sure it must be very cruel."

Joy said nothing about these unkind remarks. But she thought to herself that if the ocean had feelings, he must surely be hurt. She thought of all the nice things the ocean does for us and wished she could do something to make him feel appreciated.

Now it happened that the ocean did have feelings and that he had heard the children. And Joy's friends had indeed hurt him. But the ocean could also hear the thoughts of children, so Joy's thoughts gladdened his heart and kept him from being sad.

Joy, of course, loved the ocean. As she splashed around in the water, the ocean noticed something strange. Everywhere that Joy touched the water, the salty taste turned sweet and the coldness turned warm. And so, like everyone who saw her, the ocean fell in love with Joy. He wished he could have her for his own little girl.

After the children had gone, the ocean thought about this cheerful, pleasant little girl who turned the sea sweet and warm, and whose kindness gladdened his heart. He waited for her to return. When she didn't come back, the ocean went up farther on the sands of the beach to search for her. This was the first tide. Every day the ocean came and went, all day long, looking for Joy.

When at last she did return to the beach, the ocean roared in with a special high tide so he could be closer to her.

Again, when Joy touched the water, she sweetened the salt, warmed the coldness, and gladdened the ocean's heart. The ocean decided he did not ever want to be without this beautiful feeling. He thought that he *must* have some part of Joy with him at all times. Yet of course, he did not want to harm her.

Finally, he decided that if he took Joy's shadow, part of her could be with him always and she would be unharmed. This way, he thought, he could enjoy her sweetness, warmth, and kindness every day. And so, without her knowing it, while Joy played on the sandy beach that day, the ocean took her shadow.

How happy the ocean was! He carried Joy's shadow with him everywhere. Sometimes it could be seen in the Mediterranean Sea. Other times, sailors reported a shadow about the size of a child in the North Sea. Sharks in the Persian Gulf tried to eat the shadow. Seabirds off the South American coast wanted to race with the shadow. All the time, the ocean felt good because this shadow brought sweetness, warmth, and happiness everywhere it went.

Joy didn't realize her shadow was gone until the day after it was taken. Someone wanted to play "shadow tag." This was a favorite game with the children on sunny days. But when they ran out to play that day, they discovered that Joy had no shadow!

All the children looked where her shadow should be, but no one saw it. Joy tried placing herself in all sorts of positions between the sun and the ground. Still, she couldn't find the shadow.

Joy worried about where the shadow had gone and why. She was not as happy and carefree as she had been. Sometimes she would sit for a whole day wondering about her missing shadow. For the first time in her life, Joy was sad. Everyone else was sad, too. They missed the happiness and gaiety that Joy used to bring.

In the meantime, the shadow had traveled with the ocean everywhere. Finally, it was taken clear down to the bottom of the world.

It was a bright, sunny day in Antarctica, but it was very, very cold. Behind the ice beach stood a steep, snow-covered mountain. On the shore were several seals sleeping in the sun. Hundreds of penguins played briskly on the huge chunks of ice floating in the water near the shoreline. Thousands of other penguins strutted and chattered energetically all over the beach and the mountain. Above this beach flew dozens of tan-colored birds, the size of small turkeys. These birds were called South Polar skuas.

Even though it was noisy, due to the constant chatter of the penguins, the skuas flew along undisturbed. The big seals slept comfortably in the sun, not at all bothered by either the noise or the cold weather.

Suddenly everything grew quiet. The penguins stopped chattering. The skuas stopped flapping their wings and began gliding in to land. The seals, awakened by the silence, raised their heads and began to look around carefully.

Can you guess what happened? The animals had heard an unfamiliar noise. A tiny little voice had said, "I'm cold." The voice belonged to Joy's shadow. This was the first time a shadow ever talked.

Even though it was a weak voice, the strangeness of a child's voice made all the animals alert and attentive, since these animals had never seen a child.

When the voice came again, "Please help me, I'm cold," the animals searched for it. They found the voice and the shadow wedged between two large pieces of ice near the edge of the beach.

Several penguins helped free Joy's shadow from the ice. After the warming rays of the sun had done their work and the excited penguins had become quiet, the biggest seal spoke. "Where in the world did you come from, little shadow?" he asked.

"I belong to a little girl named Joy. And I wish I were with her right now," sobbed the shadow.

The animals understood this, of course, because they each had a shadow and knew that a shadow properly belongs to its owner. "Well, how did you ever get here?" another seal asked.

"The ocean brought me," answered the shadow, "but I'm sure Joy would like to have me back."

"Is there anything we can do to help?" a penguin inquired.

"Do you know the ocean?" asked the shadow, looking anxiously at the friendly faces.

"Oh yes, we all know him well," replied the penguin.

"Perhaps if you were to talk with him, he would agree to return me to Joy." The shadow waited for a volunteer.

Finally, the senior skua offered to carry the message to the ocean. When the ocean heard the bird's plea, he felt terrible. "I never meant to make anyone unhappy," he said. "What can I do?"

"You must see that Joy's shadow is returned," the skua said.

"I'm so ashamed," the ocean moaned, "and now Joy will hate me forever."

"Oh, I don't think so. She sounds very understanding. And besides," added the skua, "she'll be so happy to have her shadow back, she won't hate anyone!"

"But I will never be able to explain to Joy. Why, I wouldn't even be able to face her." The ocean was so sad. "Will someone else please talk to Joy for me?"

One of the penguins stepped forward. "Well, the shadow must be returned," he said, "and I've always wanted to travel, perhaps even live abroad. I'll go to Joy."

"And you'll tell her I meant no harm by taking her shadow?" the ocean asked.

"Yes," said the penguin, "I'll explain why you did it."

"And will you ask her to come to the beach and see me as often as she can?" The ocean was beginning to brighten a little.

"Yes, yes, I'll take care of it." The penguin was getting anxious to leave.

So that is how the penguin got to take his first long trip. In order to make sure it was a safe trip, the ocean gave the penguin and the shadow a special protector, one of the most ferocious animals alive—a giant killer whale.

After a safe and speedy journey, they arrived at the beach where Joy was sitting quietly and sadly alone. You can imagine how delighted Joy was to receive both her shadow and a penguin.

She forgave the ocean at once and invited the penguin to stay and live with her for as long as he wished. Of course, this was just what the penguin had wished for.

Joy became happy and gay once more. Once again everyone smiled when she smiled. Once again everything was warmer each time she laughed. And from then on, through her thoughtfulness and kindness, everything she looked upon fell in love with her, but no one ever again took her shadow.

The reason for this was the penguin! The ocean had provided a magic power to him which allowed the penguin to keep Joy's shadow forever with her. So even when Joy went to the sea, where she sweetened the salt, warmed the cold, and touched the heart of the ocean, her shadow stayed with her.

If you are so lucky as to have a penguin, take good care of it. Many people who know this story believe that all penguins—sometimes even pictures of penguins—have the power to keep your shadow attached to you. These same people believe that if you are a pretty little girl, your penguin will keep the ocean tides returning each day to look for someone to turn the salt sweet, to warm the cold, and to gladden the briny heart.

The Mule

You may have heard it said that someone is "as stubborn as a mule." This animal, a relative of the horse, has been the subject of many jokes.

One time, however, the mule was a hero. His story is told in an ancient legend about Hephaestus, the god of handicrafts and fire.

Hephaestus was the workman of the immortals who made their homes, furnishings, and weapons. He was not a handsome god and had been lame from birth. But because he was very pleasant, and moreover could make anything, he was well loved by all.

Once when Queen Hera was "as stubborn as a mule," Zeus asked Hephaestus to make something that would help the goddess be more agreeable. Zeus thought that if Hera would just sit still and think for a while, her disposition would improve.

Hephaestus thought about it and decided to make a strong invisible net to put around Hera's throne. When this was done, Hephaestus returned to his home.

Sure enough, the very first time Hera sat down on her throne, the net snapped shut and she couldn't move.

At first she was very angry. But after she sat bound in her throne for a while, thinking of why this had happened, she realized that she really must try harder to get along with people.

Finally, she called Zeus to her. "I am truly sorry that I have been so troublesome," she said. "I have been selfish and stubborn and have complained when I really had no reason. If you will free me from this invisible net, I promise I will try to keep my temper and be more cheerful and helpful."

This was exactly what Zeus had hoped for. Immediately he began to try to set Hera free. But remember, this was an invisible net, and Zeus could not find a way to break it.

All the gods and goddesses in Olympus came to help. But one by one, they gave up. No one could figure out a way to release the queen. She became frightened and began weeping. And because Hera was so unhappy, a great sadness came over everyone.

When Zeus realized that he would have to send for Hephaestus, he called on Hermes, the beautiful messenger of the gods.

It was a long journey, but you remember that Hermes had wings on his feet. Quickly he traveled down from the heavens, across the oceans, past cities and fields. At last he came to the mountains where Hephaestus lived and worked.

One of the mountains was very large and had an opening in its top through which it belched flame. The fire in it was used by Hephaestus to forge tools from metal. This was a volcano.

At the foot of the volcano, Hermes saw many elves and giants. These were the helpers of Hephaestus. They all worked together happily, singing and shouting, as they made beautiful furniture and chariots and many other lovely things. When Hermes asked for Hephaestus, he was directed up a certain path.

Suddenly he saw two huge, handsome dogs. These famous "Dogs of Hephaestus" were very clever guards. They could see inside people. If people had kind thoughts, the dogs let them pass. If their thoughts were unkind, they got no farther up the path. The dogs let Hermes pass as if they didn't even notice he was there!

Then Hermes came to a door in the side of the mountain. When he knocked, the door was opened by a beautiful maiden. She was a special maiden because she had been made from iron by Hephaestus. She did his housework and acted as his hostess.

When she took Hermes inside the mountain, he found it had been made into a beautiful home.

After the iron maiden had seated her guest, she brought refreshments of ambrosia and nectar, the favorite food and drink of the gods.

Soon Hephaestus appeared. "Greetings, gentle Hermes," he said. "Welcome to the workshop of heaven. What brings you this great distance?"

"Zeus has sent me for your help," Hermes replied. "Do you remember the invisible net you made to quiet Hera?"

"Yes, I remember," Hephaestus said with a smile. "Did it serve its purpose?"

"It served well. But when Zeus decided to set her free, no one could loosen the net. Hera is acting very nicely now, but she is still trapped in her throne. Can you come and set her free?" Hermes spoke sadly, thinking of the sadness in heaven.

"Oh, yes, I could do it in a minute," Hephaestus answered, "but it is a long journey and I am lame, as you know. I don't see how I could make that long trip in a short time."

"If I find some way to help you get to Olympus, will you come?" Hermes asked.

"Of course." And Hephaestus, sure that Hermes would find a way, began to gather his tools.

Hermes looked for some animal to carry Hephaestus. If he had been in South America, he might have found a llama. If he had been in the western part of the United States, a great mountain ram could have done the job. If he had been in Europe, the sure-footed mountain goat would have been a good choice. But Hermes searched through the mountains of Hephaestus and found only one small rabbit.

Just when Hermes was about to give up, one of the elves came by with a mule that carried food up the mountain to the workers. The mule was strong and sure-footed. Hermes had found the answer to his problem. And the mule was honored to serve a god.

So, with Hephaestus on his back, the mule was led to heaven by beautiful Hermes.

Of course, a mule had never been in heaven before, but this humble animal was welcomed by all the gods and goddesses because they were so glad to see Hephaestus. They knew he was the only one who could free their queen. Only then could they all be happy again.

So—thanks to the helpful mule—Hephaestus, the master craftsman, was able to bring laughter back to Olympus. In the twinkling of an eye, Hera was free and gloom was chased out of heaven.

The next time you see a mule, you might remember this story of the day that the mule was a hero and brought happiness to the gods.

The Cow

Did you know that according to an ancient Greek story cows were a part of the discovery of music?

Handsome Apollo was god of poetry, learning, astronomy, mathematics, medicine, and science. You can see that he was especially interested in things that made our world a better place.

Apollo was a pleasant and happy fellow who had many friends. His friends admired him because he was a hard worker and a modest god. He was modest about almost everything—with one exception. His one pride was his fine herd of cows.

These cows delighted him more than words can describe. Sometimes the other gods teased him about this one immodesty. But Apollo still spent every spare moment caring for his beloved cows.

When Apollo learned that he was going to have a baby brother, he was very happy. He thought of all the good times they would have together.

When the brother arrived, he was named Hermes.

Gods, of course, grew wise and strong very quickly. You may know the story of how Apollo killed a monster when he was only 4 days old. Hermes also grew quickly, but in his case he also became mischievous very quickly. On the very first day of his life, he decided to have an adventure. He began by telling his mother such charming stories that she fell asleep.

Then this baby god, Hermes, set off in search of mischief.

He had a marvelous time, seeing and touching all the wonders of the world.

One of the first things he found was a lovely tortoise shell. He began amusing himself by placing strings on the shell and plucking them.

The next thing he saw that interested him was a magnificent herd of cows. Just for fun—and to practice his new cleverness—he took the cows from their field and hid them, erasing their tracks so no one could find them.

He did not know whose cows they were. Do you know? Of course, they belonged to Apollo, his brother.

When Apollo discovered his herd was missing, he was angry beyond belief. When gods became angry they did terrible things. Apollo pushed down trees and tore open mountains. He even dried up rivers. But no matter how angry he became or where he looked, he could not find his cows.

Little Baby Hermes, who had hidden the cows so well, did not realize what trouble he had caused. He continued to play with his tortoise shell and string. Finally he had placed seven strings on the shell and was quite pleased with the sounds they made.

When Apollo could bear his loss no longer, he went to Zeus. "All-powerful god of gods, please help me," he begged. "My beautiful cows have disappeared. I have searched everywhere but cannot find them. I am desperate. Please, oh please, help me find my cows."

Zeus immediately called all the gods together and spoke to them. "I fear that someone has played a joke on good Apollo," he said. "Will the guilty one please come forth."

The playful 1-day-old Hermes stepped forward. "I hid the cows," he cheerfully admitted. "I didn't know they belonged to Apollo. I meant no harm. I just thought it would be fun. I'm sorry."

Apollo reached for his baby brother to spank him, but Zeus stopped him. Hermes returned the cows immediately and apologized again, but Apollo was still angry.

To calm his brother, Hermes began to pluck the seven strings on his tortoise shell. Suddenly the air was filled with beautiful melodies. This was the first music and all the gods were surprised and delighted. A great peaceful calm came over everyone—even Apollo.

"This is something I made today," Hermes said. "I have decided to call it a lyre, and the sound that comes from it will be called music. It will make people happy forever. It is a gift for you, Apollo, to show you that I am truly sorry for my mischief."

Even on Olympus, no one had ever seen such a peace offering. Apollo was deeply moved. He accepted the lyre and his brother's apology.

"I forgive you," he said with an understanding smile. As Apollo looked more closely at his wonderful gift, he said, "Tell me, Hermes, why did you choose seven strings for the lyre?"

"I put one string for each thing that you control, brother Apollo. There is one string each for poetry, learning, astronomy, mathematics, medicine, and science."

"But that is only six things," Apollo said, "and there are seven strings."

Hermes smiled. "I added the seventh," he said, "because I know that you will become such a music master that you will also become god of music."

From that day on, Apollo carried the lyre with him everywhere. Just as Hermes had predicted, Apollo played the marvelous instrument so well that he became the god of music.

The two brothers became the best of friends. Later, Hermes gave Apollo the second musical instrument. He cut reeds in the field and made the shepherd's pipes. Apollo loved and mastered this instrument also. He was known throughout Olympus for his beautiful music. The gods and goddesses spent many happy hours enjoying it. And today, music is still one of the best of all the things that people know.

So that is how our friends the cows played a part in the discovery of music. Perhaps that is why today cows are said to give more milk if their owners play soothing music for them.

Can you think of other ways that music makes our lives better?

Correspondence

Dear Ezra:

It was most considerate, thoughtful and generous of you to present me with the chocolates. Being married to a real chocoholic meant that you brought the greatest joy to our household. In addition I appreciate instruction from a continental gentleman concerning the merit of fine European chocolate.

I hope you enjoyed Christmas. There is no way I can tell you how much I appreciate your efforts to force me to organize and reflect on my life.

Take good care. We send new year tidings to all your family.

Yours in The struggle,
Chester

Letter from Chester Pierce to Ezra Griffith expressing appreciation to Griffith for his work on the biography. It marks the start of their collaboration on the project.

28 December 1995

Dear Ezra:

It was most considerate, thoughtful and generous of you to present me with the chocolates. Being married to a real chocoholic meant that you brought the greatest joy to our household. In addition I appreciate instructions from a continental gentleman concerning the merit of fine European chocolate.

I hope you enjoyed Christmas. There is no way I can tell you how much I appreciate your efforts to force me to organize and reflect on my life.

Take good care. We send New Year's tidings to all your family.

Yours in the struggle,
Chet

HARVARD MEDICAL SCHOOL HARVARD GRADUATE SCHOOL OF EDUCATION

Chester M. Pierce, M.D.
*Professor of Education
and Psychiatry in the
Faculty of Medicine and
at the Graduate School
of Education.*

Nichols House
Appian Way
Cambridge, Mass. 02138
617-495-4929

25 November 1996

Dear Ezra:

Patsy and I send our deepest sympathy to all of your family. Please tell Brigitte that both of us know, as do you, the great sorrow of losing one' mother. However, it was a blessing to have had her mother for so many years.

Words bring limited solace at a time like this, when grief is at its zenith. It goes without saying that should there be anything we can do please let us know.

The coming holidays in November and December will be burdened by the absence of mother and grandmother. Within that impossible barrier please have as comfortable time as possible.

Sincerely,
Patsy and Chet Pierce

Letter from Patsy and Chester Pierce to Ezra Griffith and his wife, Brigitte, on the occasion of the death of Brigitte's mother.

25 November 1996

Dear Ezra: Patsy and I send our deepest sympathy to all of your family. Please tell Brigitte that both of us know, as do you, the great sorrow of losing one's mother. However, it was a blessing to have had her mother for so many years.

Words bring limited solace at a time like this, when grief is at its zenith. It goes without saying that should there be anything we can do please let us know.

The coming holidays in November and December will be burdened by the absence of mother and grandmother. Within that impassable barrier please have as comfortable a time as possible.

Sincerely,

Patsy and Chet Pierce

20 March 1998

Dear Ezra:

Thank you for sustaining my "supernormal" existence. When it was time to be a Boy Scout, I was a Boy Scout. When it was time to retire. I retired.

When it was time for a biography, thanks to you, are immortalized. It was not too unseemly early, nor was it too lamentably late!

My Old Dad would demand that I show proper respect and appreciation by sending you, "a little something." I'm sure he would want something more substantive than the, literal, little something I'll dispatch. Nevertheless he may have given me some merit if he realized the gift is to insure that you won't become over extended should you have any disposable time.

Yours in the struggle,
Chet

Letter from Chester Pierce to Ezra Griffith thanking Griffith for writing _Race and Excellence_. Pierce refers to his supernormal existence (see Chapter 1) and doing things at expected stages of one's life course.

20 March 1998

Dear Ezra:

Thank you for sustaining my "supernormal" existence. When it was time to be a Boy Scout, I was a Boy Scout. When it was time to retire, I retired.

When it was time for a biography, thanks to you, one materialized. It was not too unseemly early. Nor was it too lamentably late!

My Old Dad would demand that I show proper respect and appreciation by sending you, "a little something." I'm sure he would want something more substantive than the, literal, little something I'll dispatch. Nevertheless he may have given me some merit if he realized the gift is to insure that you won't become overextended should you have any disposable time.

Yours in the struggle,
Chet

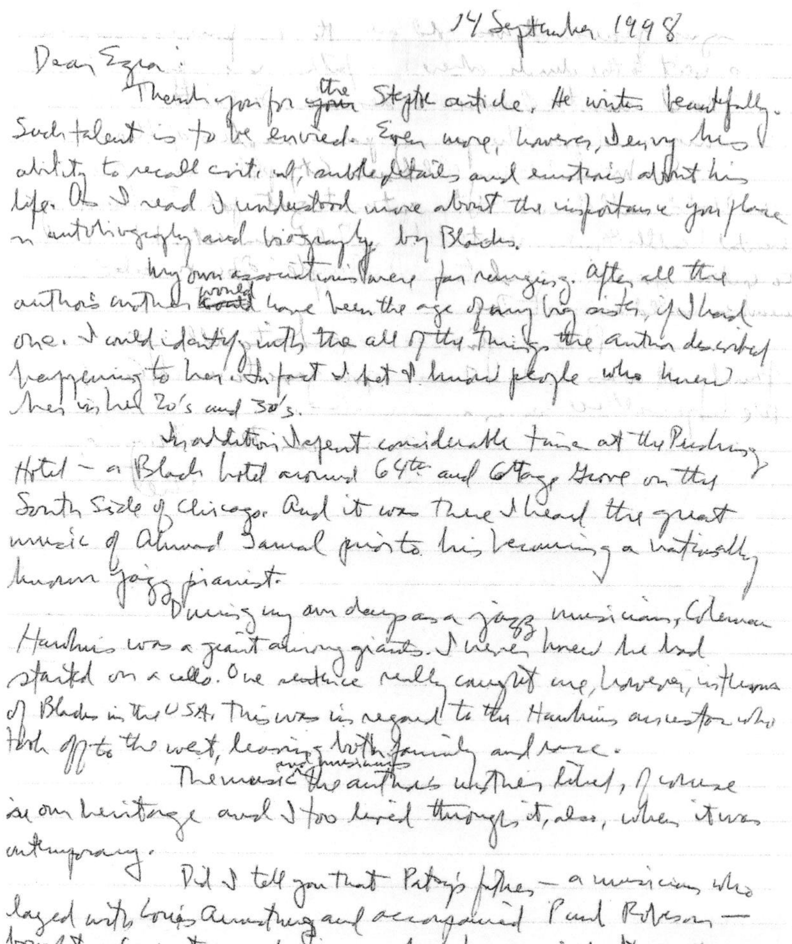

14 September 1998

Dear Ezra:

Thank you for the Stepto article. He writes beautifully. Such talent is to be envied. Even more, however, I envy his ability to recall critical, subtle details and emotions about his life. As I read I understood more about the importance you place on autobiography and biography by Blacks.

My own associations were far reaching. After all the author's mother would have been the age of my big sister, if I had one. I could identify with the all of the things the author described happening to her. In fact I bet I knew people who knew her in her 20's and 30's.

In addition I spent considerable time at the Pershing Hotel – a Black hotel around 64th and Cottage Grove on the South Side of Chicago. And it was there I heard the great music of Ahmad Jamal prior to his becoming a nationally known jazz pianist.

During my own days as a jazz musician, Coleman Hawkins was a giant among giants. I never knew he had started on a cello. One sentence really caught me, however, in terms of Blacks in the USA. This was in regard to the Hawkins ancestor who took off to the west, leaving both family and race.

The music and musicians the author's mother liked, of course is our heritage and I too lived through it, also, when it was contemporary.

Did I tell you that Patsy's father — a musician who played with Louis Armstrong and accompanied Paul Robeson — bought a concert grand piano when he married. It cost more than the house he bought in which Patsy spent her

Letter from Chester Pierce to Ezra Griffith in which Pierce references an autobiographical piece written by Robert Stepto, the John M. Schiff Professor Emeritus of English and professor of African American Studies at Yale University, about early life in Chicago. Stepto's writing leads Pierce to other memories. Pierce also mentions Gene Goold, a friend from Oklahoma. The "Apple" in the penultimate paragraph refers to the American Academy of Psychiatry and the Law, commonly known as AAPL.

growing up years. It was sold only after her parents died. The piano went to the church, where her father had been an active and beloved minister of music for decades. So ~~this to~~ This also was in my mind from the opening paragraphs of the story.

Meanwhile my Oklahoma City policeman friend, Gene Goold, called me about wanting to get police training by mental health efforts, restarted in Oklahoma City. I told him to contact you in regard to whether your "apple" office for selected members could assist them.

Please give our regards to all your family. It was such a treat you gave to us in Cambridge. We hope we'll see you in a few weeks.

Yours in the struggle,

Chet

Letter from Chester Pierce to Ezra Griffith in which Pierce references Robert Stepto, and Gene Goold (continued).

14 September 1998

Dear Ezra:

Thank you for the Stepto article. He writes beautifully. Such talent is to be envied. Even more, however, I envy his ability to recall critical, subtle details and emotions about his life. As I read it I understood more about the importance you place on autobiography and biography by Blacks.

My own associations were far ranging. After all the author's mother would have been the age of my big sister, if I had one. I could identify with all of the things the author described happening to her. In fact I bet I knew people who knew her in her 20's and 30's.

In addition I spent considerable time at the Pershing Hotel—a Black hotel around 64th and Cottage Grove on the South Side of Chicago. And it was there I heard the great music of Ahmad Jamal prior to his becoming a nationally known jazz pianist.

During my own days as a jazz musician, Coleman Hawkins was a giant among giants. I never knew he had started on a cello. One sentence really caught me, however, is the one of Blacks in the USA. This was in regard to the Hawkins ancestor who took off to the West, leaving both family and race.

The music and musicians the author's mother liked, of course are our heritage and I too lived through it, also, when it was contemporary.

Did I tell you that Patsy's father—a musician who played with Louis Armstrong and accompanied Paul Robeson—bought a concert grand piano when he married. It cost more than the house he bought in which Patsy spent her growing up years. It was sold only after her parents died. The piano went to the church where her father had been an active and beloved minister of music for decades. So all this also was in mind from the opening paragraphs of the story.

Meanwhile my Oklahoma City policeman friend, Gene Goold, called me about wanting to get police training, by mental health experts, restarted in Oklahoma City. I told him to contact you in regard to whether the "Apple" office or selected members could assist them.

Please give our regards to all your family. It was such a treat you gave to us in Cambridge. We hope we'll see you in a few weeks.

Yours in the struggle,
Chet

5 October 1998

Dear Ezra:

    As you see this more and more casual about attending to thank you note. It seems that time is passing more fast than it used did — and I seem to be able to get less and less done — all the while, while I seem to be doing nothing at all.

    Thanks for the stirring tribute you did about Charley. It was a wonderful piece.

    I saw Alan Stone and we chatted about your article. He seemed very pleased that you had written it and of course he talked about the impact his decision about the Sergeant had on his life.

    A couple of people have told me they saw a review of your book in JAMA. I assume it was

Letter from Chester Pierce to Ezra Griffith in which reference is made to Charles Pinderhughes, a former Tufts University professor and psychoanalyst, and to Alan Stone, Touroff-Glueck Professor of Law and Psychiatry Emeritus at Harvard University. "Carl" refers to Carl Bell, who was a professor of psychiatry and public health at the University of Illinois, Chicago.

they were inspired to buy a copy.

Parents day is almost here. Let us know when you are coming and when you'll be free to go to dinner. Even though he's a struggling pensioner, my old dad can afford to take your family and you to a place where the patrons can appreciate a Paris wardrobe!

I know you are busy doing all manner of things. Further I know you are doing them thoughtfully and well. I look forward to seeing you soon. Patsy and I send our warmest regards to all of you.

Yours in the struggle,
Chet

Letter from Chester Pierce to Ezra Griffith in which reference is made to Charles Pinderhughes and Alan Stone *(continued).*

5 October 1998

Dear Ezra:

As you see I'm more and more casual about attending to thank you notes. It seems that time is passing more fast than it ever did—and I seem to be able to get less and less done—all the while, while I seem to be doing nothing at all.

Thanks for the stirring tribute you did about Charley. It was a wonderful piece.

I saw Alan Stone and we chatted about your article. He seemed very pleased that you had written it and of course he talked about the impact his decision about the sergeant had on his life.

A couple of people have told me they saw a review of your book in JAMA. I assume it was the one you told me Carl was doing. At any rate they were inspired to buy a copy.

Parents Day is almost here. Let us know when you are coming and when you'd be free to go to dinner. Even though I am a struggling pensioner, my old dad can afford to take your family and you to a place where the patrons can appreciate a Paris wardrobe!

I know you are busy doing all manner of things. Further I know you are doing them thoroughly and well. I look forward to seeing you soon. Patsy and I send our earnest regards to all of you.

Yours in the struggle,
Chet

6 August 2007

Dear Ezra:

Only a few days ago did I
learn of your recent APA honor.
Please accept my sincere, if belated,
congratulations. Indeed you have had
a distinguished career and the
organization honors itself by
honoring you.

I hope this note finds your
family and you in the best of health
and spirit. All of you stay in our
prayers, especially Veronique.

Letter from Chester Pierce to Ezra Griffith. This is the first time Pierce does not sign off with his usual "yours in the struggle."

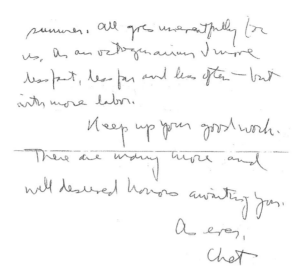

Letter from Chester Pierce to Ezra Griffith in which Pierce does not sign off with his usual "yours in the struggle" *(continued).*

6 August 2007

Dear Ezra:

Only a few days ago did I learn of your recent APA honor. Please accept my sincere, if belated, congratulations. Indeed you have had a distinguished career and the organization honors itself by honoring you.

I hope this note finds your family and you in the best of health and spirit. All of you stay in our prayers, especially Véronique.

Meanwhile enjoy the summer. All goes uneventfully for us. As an octogenarian I move less fast, less far and less often—but with more labor.

Keep up your good work. There are many more and well deserved honors awaiting you.

As ever,
Chet

Poem Letter by Richard Fournier, L.C.S.W., May 4, 1998

Dear Ezra,
 Probably, Dear Chester,
Not clear where one leaves off,
The other rushes in to celebrate:
 the connection,
 the mentoring,
 the nurturing,
 the chaste fertilization,
 the admiration,
 the love and devotion.

Intelligence, charm, frequent wit,
Self-conscious wit, even French a bit;
Dangerously modest, discreet and silent;
Sometimes anesthetized by the limits of
Pained injustice and Racism's venom.
"Written with grace and conviction."
The closest you'll probably ever come
 to letting the world see with what
 intimacy and courage you can love.
Paranoia and prudence are, indeed, a
 basket under which to hide
 even the most radiant of candles.

From the resigned, but true
"Parents can buy the machete
 and pay for the instruction..."
  to the
 "exotic" and "mundane environment,"
 the compelling, exquisitely committed,
  emergent commitments
 shine through a fine and subtle patina:
"The love of anonymity dictates much of what we do."
Indeed, this is quiet excellence;
 reserved distinction.
But then again,
That's you!

Celebration of Life

A MEMORIAL CELEBRATION
FOR THE LIFE OF

CHESTER M. PIERCE
MARCH 4, 1927 - SEPTEMBER 23, 2016

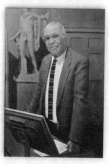

FRIDAY, SEPTEMBER 22, 2017
1:00 PM

Memorial Church

HARVARD UNIVERSITY
ONE HARVARD YARD
CAMBRIDGE, MA

Welcome

David Henderson, MD
Professor and Chair of Psychiatry
Boston University School of Medicine

Remarks

Jerrold Rosenbaum, MD
Psychiatrist-in-Chief, MGH
Stanley Cobb Professor of Psychiatry,
Harvard Medical School

Elliot Sorel, MD, DLFAPA
Senior Scholar for Healthcare Innovations,
Clinical Professor of Global Health,
George Washington University

Altha Stewart, MD
President-Elect
American Psychiatric Association

Ezra Griffith, MD
Professor Emeritus of Psychiatry,
Yale School of Medicine

Miguel Williams *(grandson)*

John Williams *(Son-in-law)*

Reception to Follow - Harvard Faculty Club
(map on reverse of program)

Publications by
Chester Middlebrook Pierce

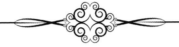

Books

Bedau H, Pierce CM (eds): Capital Punishment in the United States. New York, AMS Press, 1976

Kales A, Pierce CM, Greenblatt M (eds): The Mosaic of Contemporary Psychiatry in Perspective. New York, Springer-Verlag, 1991

Mathis JL, Pierce CM, Pishkin V: Basic Psychiatry, 2nd Edition. New York, Appleton-Century-Crofts, 1971 (Japanese edition 1978)

Pierce CM: The Shell Fairy: A Children's Operetta. Adapted by S Beattie; music by Anderson TJ (unpublished), 1977

Pierce CM (ed): Television and Behavior. Beverly Hills, CA, Sage, 1978

Articles

Brooks RE, Natani K, Shurley JT, et al: A South Polar sleep and dream laboratory. Psychophysiology 7:356, 1970

Cobb A, Main, RL, Pierce CM: Barriers in pastoral counseling research. Ment Hyg 49:337–340, 1965 14313921

Dalrymple S, Pierce CM, Bratzman E, et al: Implications of a study in nurse-physician relationships. Nursing Forum 7:21–27, 1968

Dimsdale JE, Pierce CM, Schoenfeld D, et al: Suppressed anger and blood pressure: the effects of race, sex, social class, obesity, and age. Psychosom Med 48(6):430–436, 1986 3749420

Greenblatt M, Carew J, Pierce CM: Success rates in psychiatry and neurology certification exams. Am J Psychiatry 134(11):1259–1261, 1977 910978

Guenter CA, Joern AT, Shurley JT, Pierce CM: Cardiorespiratory and metabolic effects in men on the South Polar Plateau. Arch Intern Med 125:630–637, 1970 5265836

Hofling CK, Bratzman E. Dalrymple S, et al: An experimental study in nurse-physician relationships. J Nerv Ment Dis 143(2):171–180, 1966 5957275

Joern AT, Shurley JT, Guenter CA, et al: Nocturnal sleep patterns during acute exposure to high-altitude hypoxia. Psychophysiology 7:356, 1970

Joern AT, Shurley JT, Brooks RE, et al: Short-term changes in sleep patterns on arrival at South Polar Plateau. Arch Intern Med 125(4):649–654, 1970 4314525

Lipcon HH, Pierce CM: Somnambulism: electroencephalographic studies and related findings. US Armed Forces Med J 7(10):1419–1426, 1956 13392145

Lipcon HH, Pierce CM: Clinical relationship of enuresis to sleep-walking and epilepsy. AMA Arch Neurol Psychiatry 76(3):310–316, 1956 13354052

Lipcon HH, McLary JH, Noble HF, Pierce CM: Enuresis: psychiatric interview studies. US Armed Forces Med J 7(9):1265–1280, 1956 13361108

Mathis JL, Lester BK, Pierce CM: A method for serial sampling of blood during sleep. Am J Psychiatry 118:249–250, 1961 13768125

Mathis JL, Pierce CM, Pishkin V: An experiment in programmed teaching of psychiatry. Am J Psychiatry 122(9):937–404, 1965 5902506

Mathis JL, Pierce CM, Lester BK: Cholesterol levels during sleep and dreams. Am J Psychiatry 124(3):389–390, 1967 6039996

Mayes N, Coles MN, Pierce CM: Commitment to nursing—how is it achieved? Nurs Outlook 16(7):29–31, 1968 5186673

Muchmore HG, Blackburn AB, Shurley JT, et al: Neutropenia in healthy men at the South Polar Plateau. Arch Intern Med 125(4):646–648, 1970 5437889

Natani K, Shurley JT, Pierce CM, Brooks RE: Long-term changes in sleep patterns in men on the South Polar Plateau. Arch Intern Med 125(4):655–659, 1970 4314526

Nixon OL, Pierce CM, Lester B, Mathis JL: Narcolepsy 1: nocturnal dream frequency in adolescents. J Neuropsychiatr, 5:150–152, 1964 14118068

Pierce CM: Brief psychotherapy on guards at a naval brig. J Soc Ther 4:41–47, 1958

Pierce CM: The recruit prisoner. Mil Med 124(2):131–140, 1959 13632434

Pierce CM: A psychiatric approach to present-day racial problems. J Natl Med Assoc 51(3):207–210, 1959 13655083

Pierce CM: Some psychiatric considerations in coaching football. J Okla State Med Assoc 53:753–759, 1960 13735533

Pierce CM: The combination of inferior dentition and psychiatric maladjustment in naval recruits. Q Natl Dent Assoc 18:63–66, 1960

Pierce CM: Psychiatric aspects of police-community relations. Ment Hyg 46:107–115, 1962 14486449

Pierce CM: Dream studies in enuresis research. Can J Psychiatr Assoc J 8:415–419, 1963 14102060

Pierce CM: Some "teachable" aspects of interviewing. J Okla State Med Assoc 56:570–577, 1963 14086195

Pierce CM: Greek poetry and modern psychotherapy. Am J Psychother 17:631–640, 1963 14060044

Pierce CM: Through Egypt with Herodotus. Medical Opinion and Review 1:57–61, 1966

Pierce CM: The dinner seminar in a program for general practitioners. South Med J 59(10):1184–1186, 1966 5925410

Pierce CM: Violence and the American character structure. Medical Opinion and Review, 3:100–109, 1967

Pierce CM: Psychiatric teaching in a general hospital. Compr Psychiatry 9:258, 1968

Pierce CM: Possible social science contributions to the clarification of the Negro self-image. J Natl Med Assoc 60(2):100–103, 1968 5649259

Pierce CM: Manpower: the need for Negro psychiatrists. J Natl Med Assoc 60:23–33, 1968

Pierce CM: Violence and counterviolence: the need for a children's domestic exchange. Am J Orthopsychiatry 39(4):553–568, 1969 5803594

Pierce CM: Our most crucial domestic issue. Am J Psychiatry 125(11):1583–1584, 1969 5776868

Pierce CM: Research and careers for blacks. Am J Psychiatry 127(6):817-818, 1970 5482876

Pierce CM: Black psychiatry one year after Miami. J Natl Med Assoc 62(6):471–473, 1970 5493608

Pierce CM: Xenophobes or cosmopolites? Am J Orthopsychiatry, 40:560–561, 1970

Pierce CM: Effect of fatigue and mental stress on football performance, in Football Injuries. National Academy of Sciences Workshop, Washington, DC, pp 205–210, 1970

Pierce CM: Some comments on educational television. U.S. Senate Select Committee on Equal Educational Opportunity, July 30: pp 928a–m, 1970

Pierce CM: The preschooler and the future. Futurist 6:13–15, 1972

Pierce CM: On food and dreams. The Academy, May 1972

Pierce CM: On becoming a planetary citizen: a quest for meaning. Childhood Education 49:5–63, 1972

Pierce CM: Drugs and public policy: pushing us towards a police state. Am J Orthopsychiatry 43(4):528–530, 1973 4716669

Pierce CM: Television, behavior modification, and fetal tissue procurement: the impact and challenge to Black women. Binding Ties, 2:19–24, 1974

Pierce CM, Allen G: Childism. Psychiatr Ann 5:15–24, 1975

Pierce CM: A report on minority children. Psychiatr Ann 5:60–84, 1975

Pierce CM: The ghetto: an extreme sleep environment. J Natl Med Assoc 67(2):162–166, 1975 1133867

Pierce CM: Capital punishment: effects of the death penalty: data and deliberations from the social sciences. Am J Orthopsychiatry, 45(4):580, 1975 1180341

Pierce CM: Some comments on Defunis. Black Law Journal, 4:277–281, 1975

Pierce CM: Football: the psychology of competition, in Five Minute Hour. Ardsley, NY, Geigy Pharmaceuticals, 1976

Pierce CM: Television and education. Education and Urban Society 10:3–9, 1977

Pierce CM: Entitlement dysfunctions. Aust NZJ Psychiatry 12(4):215–219, 1978 283790

Pierce CM: Twenty-first century orthopsychiatry: extragalactic to submolecular concerns. Am J Orthopsychiatry 54(3):364–368, 1984 6465289

Pierce CM: Television and violence: social psychiatric perspectives. Am J Soc Psychiatry 4:41–44, 1984

Pierce CM: Social science research in high latitudes. J Clin Psychol 41:5–81, 1985

Pierce CM: Mental health factors in spaceflight. Aviat Space Environ Med 59(2):99–101, 1988 3345184

Pierce CM: Ecology and mental health. J Clin Psychol 50(1):110–111, 1994 8150990

Pierce CM: Joe Yamamoto, M. D., president 1994–1995. Am J Orthopsychiatry, 64:338–340, 1994

Pierce CM: Ezra Griffith, president 1997–1998. Am J Orthopsychiatry, 67:338–340, 1997

Pierce CM, Dickerson R: The occupational therapy shop as a culture: theoretical considerations. Am J Occup Ther 16:231–235, 1962 14486448

Pierce CM, Gool JE: Collaboration in the protection of a president. Correct Soc Psych J Behav Tech Methods Ther 10:331–338, 1964

Pierce CM, Lipcon HH: Somnambulism: psychiatric interview studies. US Armed Forces Med J 7(8):1143–1153, 1956 13352553

Pierce CM, Lipcon HH: Aids in the diagnosis of epilepsy in service men. Dis Nerv Syst 20:342–345, 1959

Pierce CM, Lipcon HH: A survey of bedwetting. South Med J 52:1520–1524, 1959 14432818

Pierce CM, Lipcon HH: Stuttering: clinical and electroencephalographic findings. Mil Med 124(7):511–519, 1959

Pierce CM, Shurley JT: Current status of medical research in American bases in Antarctica. Antarctica Journal, 167, 1968

Pierce CM, West LJ: Six years of sit-ins: psychodynamic causes and effects. Int J Soc Psychiatry 12(1):29–34, 1966 5906140

Pierce CM, Lipcon HH, McLary JH, Noble HF: Enuresis: clinical, laboratory, and electroencephalographic studies. US Armed Forces Med J 7(2):208–219, 1956 13291594

Pierce CM, Whitman R, Maas J, Gay M: Enuresis and dreaming: experimental studies. Arch Gen Psychiatry 4:166–170, 1961 13735532

Pierce CM, West LJ, Thomas WD: Of elephants and psychiatry. Proceedings of the Midwestern Zoological Society, 1963

Pierce CM, Downing MJ, DeBroux K: Why a nurse in a day treatment center? Ment Hosp 15:446–447, 1964

Pierce CM, Mathis JL, Lester BK, Nixon OL: Dreams of food during sleep experiments. Psychosomatics 5:374–377, 1964

Pierce CM, Schwartz D Thomas EM: Music therapy in a day care center. Dis Nerv Syst 25:29–32, 1964 14105067

Pierce CM, Mathis JL, Jabbour JT: Dream patterns in narcoleptic and hydrancephalic patients. Am J Psychiatry 122(4):402–404, 1965 5890011

Pierce CM, Mathis JL, Pishkin V: Basic psychiatry in twelve hours: (an experiment in programmed learning) Dis Nerv Syst 29(8):533–535, 1968 5677253

Pierce CM, Manglesdorf, T, Whitman, R. M. Mothers of enuretic boys. Am J Psychother 23:283–292, 1969

Pierce CM, Carew J, Pierce-Gonzalez D, Wills D: An experiment in racism: TV commercials. Education and Urban Society 10:61–87, 1977

Pierce CM, Stillner V, Popkin M: On the meaning of sports: cross cultural observations of super stress. Cult Med Psychiatry 6(1):11–28, 1982 7105786

Pishkin V, Pierce CM, Mathis JL: Analysis of attitudinal and personality variables in relation to a programmed course in psychiatry. J Clin Psychol 23(1):52–56, 1967 4382194

Popkin M, Stillner V, Osborne LW, et al: Novel behaviors in an extreme environment. Am J Psychiatry 131(6):651–654, 1974 4133304

Popkin M, Stillner V, Pierce CM, et al: Recent life changes and outcome of prolonged competitive stress. J Nerv Ment Dis 163(5):302–306, 1976 978186

Popkin MK, Pierce CM, Stillner V: The Iditarod: Alaskan challenge. Phys Sportsmed 5(3):78–84, 1977 27399187

Popkin MK, Hall RC, Stillner V, Pierce CM: A generalized response to protracted stress? Mil Med, 143(7):479–480, 1978 97593

Popkin MK, Stillner V, Eckman J, et al: Blood changes in men stressed by a 1049-mile sled-dog race. Alaska Med, 22(3):33–39, 1980 7190781

Popkin M, Pierce CM, Stillner V, et al: Hematological changes with prolonged competitive stress in the North. Moscow, Izdatelstvo Medisina, 1980

Popkin M, Stillner V, Pierce CM, Organic mental disorder associated with prolonged competitive stress. Compr. Psychiatry, 22:522–527, 1981

Rimel WM, Pierce CM: A peregrinating problem patient: (psychiatric case study of Munchausen's syndrome). Dis Nerv Syst 22:139–144, 1961 13741708

Ryan AJ, Ogilvie BC, Morgan WC, et al: The emotionally disturbed athlete. The Physician and Sportsmedicine 7:66–80, 1981

Shannon J, Kaplan SM, Pierce CM, Ross WD: An interesting reaction to a tranquilizer: tonic seizures with perphenazine (Trilafon). Am J Psychiatry 114(6):556, 1957 13478778

Shurley JT, Pierce CM, Natani K, Brooks RE: Sleep and activity patterns at South Pole Station: a preliminary report. Arch Gen Psychiatry 22(5):385–389, 1970 5436864

Stillner V, Popkin MK, Pierce CM: Caffeine-induced delirium during prolonged competitive stress. Am J Psychiatry 135(7):855–856, 1978 665803

Stillner V, Popkin MK, Pierce CM: Biobehavioral changes in prolonged competitive stress. Med Sci Sport 11:104, 1979

Stillner V, Popkin M, Pierce CM: Biobehavioral changes in prolonged competitive stress: observations of Iditarod trail sled dog mushers. Alaska Med 24(1):1–6, 1982 7091584

Stillner V, Popkin M, Pierce CM: Predicting successful athletic behavior: indicators in an athletic contest. Mil Med 148 (8):668–672, 1983 6415523

West LJ, Pierce CM, Thomas WD: Lysergic acid diethylamide: its effects on a male Asiatic elephant. Science,138(3545):1110–1113 1962 17772968

Whitcomb WH, Joern AT, Guenter CA, et al: Effect of the South Polar Plateau on plasma and urine erythropoietin levels. Arch Intern Med 125(4):638–645, 1970 5461867

Whitman RM, Pierce CM, Maas, JW, Baldridge BJ: Drugs and dreams II: imipramine and prochlorperazine. Compr Psychiatry 2:219–226, 1961 14006636

Whitman RM, Pierce CM, Maas JW, Baldridge BJ: Dreams of the experimental subject. J Nerv Ment Dis 134:431–439, 1962 14006637

Chapters

Brooks RE, Natani K, Shurley JT, et al: An Antarctic sleep and dream laboratory, in Human Polar Biology. Edited by Edholm OG, Gunderson EKE. Portsmouth, NH, William Heinemann Medical Books, 1975

Ewalt JR, Pierce CM: Commentaries on neighborhood psychiatry, in Neighborhood Psychiatry. Edited by Macht L, Scherl D, Sharfenstein S. Lexington, MA, DC Heath, 1977

Mathis JL, Pierce CM, Pishkin V: A completed psychiatric program, in Individualized Instruction in Medical Education. Edited by Lysaught JP. Rochester, NY, Rochester Clearing House, 1967

Pierce CM: Enuresis, in Comprehensive Textbook of Psychiatry. Edited by Freedman AM, Kaplan HL. Baltimore, MD, Williams and Wilkins, 1966

Pierce CM: Life sciences in 2040 A.D., in The World of Ideas: Essays on the Past and Future. Edited by Cross GL. Norman, University of Oklahoma Press, 1968

Pierce CM: Problems of the Negro adolescent in the next decade, in Minority Group Adolescents in the U.S. Edited by Brody E. Baltimore, MD, William and Wilkins, 1968

Pierce CM: Is bigotry the basis of the medical problems in the ghetto?, in Medicine in the Ghetto. Edited by Norman JC. New York, Appleton-Century-Crofts, 1969

Pierce CM: Offensive mechanisms, in The Black Seventies. Edited by Barbout F. Boston, MA, Porter Sargent, 1970

Pierce CM: Mental readiness for competition, in Fundamentals of Athletic Training: A Manual on Athletic Training Published Under the Joint Auspices of the AMA's Committee on the Medical Aspects of Sports, the National Athletic Trainers Association, and the Athletic Institute. Chicago, IL, American Medical Association, 1971

Pierce CM, Relevance of Antarctic biomedical research to society in the 70's, in Proceedings of Colloquium on Polar Medicine. Washington, DC, National Academy of Sciences, National Research Council, 1971

Pierce CM: The formation of the Black Psychiatrists of America, in Racism and Mental Health. Edited by Willie CV, Kramer BM, Brown BS. Pittsburgh, PA, University of Pittsburgh, 1973

Pierce CM: Race, deprivation, and drug abuse in the U.S.A., in Proceedings of the Anglo-American Conference on Drug Abuse. London, Royal Society of Medicine, 1973

Pierce CM: Psychiatric problems of the black minority, in American Handbook of Psychiatry, Vol 2. Edited by Caplan G. New York, Basic Books, 1974

Pierce CM: Poverty and racism as they affect children, in Advocacy for Child Mental Health. Edited by Berlin I. New York, Brunner/Mazel, 1975

Pierce CM: Enuresis and encopresis, in Comprehensive Textbook of Psychiatry, 2nd Edition. Edited by Freedman AM, Kaplan HI, Sadock, BJ. Baltimore, MD, Williams and Wilkins, 1975

Pierce CM: Other special symptoms, in Comprehensive Textbook of Psychiatry, 2nd Edition. Edited by Freedman AM, Kaplan HI, Sadock BJ. Baltimore, MD, Williams and Wilkins, 1975

Pierce CM: The mundane extreme environment and its effect on learning, in Learning Disabilities: Issues and Recommendations for Research. Edited by Brainard SG. Washington, DC, National Institute of Education, Department of Health, Education and Welfare, 1975

Pierce CM: Teaching cross-racial therapy, in Working Papers of the 1975 Conference on Education of Psychiatrists. Washington, DC, American Psychiatric Association, 1976

Pierce CM: Personality disorders, in Psychiatry in General Medical Practice. Edited by Usdin G, Lewis J. New York, Blaikston, McGraw-Hill, 1979

Pierce CM, Sports and TV awareness, in Television Awareness. Edited by Moody K. New York, Media for Action Research Center, 1979

Pierce CM: Enuresis, in Comprehensive Textbook of Psychiatry, 3rd Edition. Edited by Kaplan H, Freedman A, Sadock B. Baltimore, MD, Williams and Wilkins, 1980

Pierce CM: Encopresis, in Comprehensive Textbook of Psychiatry, 3rd Edition. Edited by Kaplan H, Freedman A, Sadock B. Baltimore, MD, Williams and Wilkins, 1980

Pierce CM: Nail biting, thumb sucking, in Comprehensive Textbook of Psychiatry, 3rd Edition. Edited by Kaplan H, Freedman A, Sadock B. Baltimore, MD, Williams and Wilkins, 1980

Pierce CM: Sports and psychiatry, in Comprehensive Textbook of Psychiatry, 3rd Edition. Edited by Kaplan H, Freedman A, Sadock B. Baltimore, MD, Williams and Wilkins, 1980

Pierce CM: Social trace contaminants: subtle indicators of racism, in Television and Social Behavior: Beyond Violence and Children. Edited by Withey S, Abeles R. Hillsdale, NJ, Lawrence Erlbaum, 1980

Pierce CM: The social role of psychiatry: a look forward to the 80's, in Psychiatry in Crisis. Edited by Hall RCW. New York: Spectrum, 1982

Pierce CM: Mental health and social development, in Mental Health, Cultural Values and Social Development. Edited by Nunn RC, Butt DS, Ladrigo-Ignacio L. Dordrecht, The Netherlands: D. Reidel, 1984

Pierce CM: The handicapped, in Mental Health, Cultural Values and Social Development. Edited by Nunn RC, Butt DS, Ladrigo-Ignacio L. Dordrecht, The Netherlands, D. Reidel, 1984

Pierce CM: Other developmental disorders, in Comprehensive Psychiatry IV, Vol 2. Edited by Kaplan H, Sadock B. Baltimore, MD, Williams and Wilkins, 1985

Pierce CM: Medical philosophy and medical advocacy, in Advocacy and Anthropology. Edited by Paine R. St. John's, NL, Canada, Institute of Social and Economic Research, Memorial University of Newfoundland, 1985

Pierce CM: Enuresis, in Comprehensive Psychiatry IV, Vol 2. Edited by Kaplan H, Sadock B. Baltimore, MD, Williams and Wilkins, 1985

Pierce CM: Encopresis, in Comprehensive Psychiatry IV, Vol 2. Edited by Kaplan H, Sadock B. Baltimore, MD, Williams and Wilkins, 1985

Pierce CM: Stress in the workplace, in Black Families in Crisis. Edited by Coner-Edwards AF, Spurlock J. New York, Brunner/Mazel, 1988

Pierce CM: Impact of society on children: television as a socializing agent, in Proceedings of the Inaugural Annual Meeting, Melbourne, VIC, Australia, Faculty of Child Psychiatry, Royal Australian and New Zealand College of Psychiatrists, 1988

Pierce CM: Unity in diversity: thirty-three years of stress, in Psychosocial Issues and Academic Achievement. Edited by Berry GL, Asamen JK. Newbury Park, CA, Sage, 1989

Pierce CM: Psychiatric aspects of sports neurology, in Sports Neurology. Edited by Jordan B, Tsairis P, Warren R. Rockville, MD, Aspen, 1989

Pierce CM: Racial perspectives on the past and future, in Mosaic of Contemporary Psychiatry in Perspective. Edited by Kales A, Pierce C, and Greenblatt M. New York: Springer-Verlag, 1992

Pierce CM: Enuresis, in Psychiatry: A World Perspective, Vol 1. Edited by Stefanis CN, Rabavilas AD, Soldatos CR. Amsterdam, Excepta Medica, 1990

Pierce CM: Theoretical approaches to adaptation to Antarctica and space, in From Antarctica to Outer Space: Life in Isolation and Confinement. Edited by Harrison AA, Clearwater Y. New York, Springer-Verlag, 1991

Pierce CM: Concerning an aging psychiatrist, in How Psychiatrists Look at Aging. Edited by Pollock GH. Madison, WI, International Universities Press, 1992

Pierce CM: Mankind in space, in Social Psychiatry and World Accords. Edited by Masserman JH. New York, Gardner, 1992

Pierce CM: Stress analogs of racism and sexism: terrorism, torture and disaster, in Mental Health, Racism, and Sexism. Edited by Willie C, Rieker P, Kramer B, and Brown B. Pittsburgh, PA: University of Pittsburgh Press, 1995

Pierce CM, Kuehnle K: Neuropsychiatric aspects, in Sports and the Athletic Female. Edited by Haycock C. Oradell, NJ, Medical Economics Books, 1980

Pierce CM, Profit, WE: Homoracial and heteroracial behavior in the United States, in Mental Health in Africa and the Americas Today. Edited by Okpaku SO. Nashville, TN, Chrisolith, 1991

Pierce CM, Stuart, HJ: Mental readiness in sports, in Proceedings of the AMA Seventh National Conference on Medical Aspects of Sports. Philadelphia, PA, American Medical Association, 1967

Pierce CM, Pishkin V, Mathis JL: Some problems in developing a psychiatric program, in Programmed Instruction in Medical Education. Edited by Lysaught JP. Rochester, NY, Rochester Clearing House, 1965

Pierce CM, Earls, FJ, Kleinman A: Race and culture in psychiatry, in Handbook of Harvard Psychiatry, 3rd Edition. Edited by Nicholi A. Cambridge, MA, Harvard University Press, 1995

Ryan HH, Pierce CM, Ham TH: Report of the Subcommittee on Teaching Methods and Materials, in Teaching Psychiatry in Medical School. Washington, DC, American Psychiatric Association, 1969

Whitman RM, Pierce CM, Maas JW: Drugs and dreams, in Drugs and Behavior. Edited by Uhr L, Miller JG. New York, Wiley, 1960

Wurtzel A, Lometti G, Chaffee S., et al: The television violence-viewer debate, in The Media and Criminal Justice Policy: Recent Research and Social Efforts. Edited by Surette R. Springfield, IL, CE Thomas, 1990

Special Reports

American Public Health Association: The National Arctic Health Service Policy. American Public Health Association Report Series. Washington, DC, American Public Health Association, 1984

Commission on Engineering and Technical Systems Staff: Space Station Engineering Design Issues. Washington, DC, National Academies Press, 1989

Committee on Arctic Research Policy; Policy Research Board; Commission on Physical Sciences, Mathematics, and Resources; National

Research Council: A United States Commitment to Arctic Research. Washington, DC, National Academies Press, 1982

Hamburg BA, Pierce CM: Television and health: introductory comments, in Television and Behavior: Ten Years of Scientific Progress and Implications for the Eighties, Vol 2, Technical Reviews. DHHS Pub No (ADM) 82-1196. Washington, DC, U.S. Department of Health and Human Services, 1982

Physicians for Human Rights: Human Rights on Hold: A Report on Emergency Measures and Access to Health Care in the Occupied Territories, 1990–1992. Boston, MA, Physicians for Human Rights, 1993

Pierce C (chair): A Report to the Multicultural Task Force. Washington, DC, National Institute of Education, 1975

Pierce C (chair): Polar Biomedical Research: An Assessment. Washington, DC, National Academies Press, 1982

Pierce CM: The Future of Education. Redmond, Lake Washington School District, 1983

Pierce CM: Foreword, in Franz Fanon and the Psychology of Oppression. Bulham HA. New York, Plenum Press, 1985

Pierce C (chair): Data Coordination and Career Stimulation in Polar Biomedical Research. Washington, DC, National Academies Press, 1988

Pierce C (chair): The Arctic Aeromedical Laboratory's Thyroid Function Studies: A Radiological Risk and Ethical Analysis. Washington, DC, National Academies Press, 1996